Understanding Mechanisms of Change in Psychotherapies for Personality Disorders

Beautifully integrating research findings with rich case examples, this engaging book yields clinically relevant, actionable principles to guide therapists as they navigate critical choice points in treatment. The respectful way in which the three authors reflect on their own and each other's approaches is an exemplary model of the kind of nuanced, thoughtful dialogue that can move the field of psychotherapy forward.

—**Catherine F. Eubanks, PhD,** Professor, Gordon F. Derner School of Psychology, Adelphi University, Garden City, NY, United States

This book provides a clinically sophisticated and empirically sound overview of the treatment for personality disorders. It goes beyond the knee-jerk selection of a treatment package for a diagnostic category. Instead, it provides transtheoretical ways of personalizing the intervention with sound case formulation. What is particularly unique is that the authors go from the therapist's goals, to interventions to achieve these goals, then to the change processes that are behind these interventions. This is a major contribution to the field as few, if any, therapy guidelines with this population have presented this conceptualization. This could turn out to be a classic in the field—the go-to book on treating personality disorders.

—**Marvin R. Goldfried, PhD,** Distinguished Professor of Clinical Psychology, Stony Brook University, Stony Brook, NY, United States

Great gains have been made in developing effective psychotherapies for personality disorders. What we still don't know is how and why these therapies work. In this cleverly organized and clearly written book, Kramer and colleagues provide an essential and stimulating synthesis of the most important mechanisms of change in psychotherapy for personality disorders. It is a must-read for clinicians wanting to better articulate their impact, and for researchers wishing to track it more precisely.

—**Carla Sharp, PhD,** John and Rebecca Moores Professor; Associate Dean for Faculty and Research, CLASS; and Director of the Developmental Psychopathology Lab and ADAPT clinic, University of Houston, Houston, TX, United States

This book represents an important advance in the treatment of personality disorders: the movement beyond narrow adherence to particular "brand-name" therapies. The authors—all leading figures in personality disorder treatment and research—describe their understanding of how therapy can best work for particular patients from three distinct theoretical orientations, focusing on several important domains of functioning and moving between different levels of evidence. Through detailed clinical case examples, the authors show how various theoretical and evidence-based perspectives can converge and complement one another to maximize benefit for the individual patient. This is essential reading for any clinician who wants to become more effective in their work with patients who suffer from personality disorders. The authors address a wide range of clinical challenges and walk the reader through their thinking in how to proceed, focusing on core principles and mechanisms of change at every turn. Both early-career and seasoned clinicians will appreciate this accessible window into the therapeutic process. Moreover, the book provides a sophisticated, evidence-based rationale for long-held clinical wisdom: that psychotherapy works best when therapists can integrate from different models and personalize their interventions to the individual patient.

—**David Kealy, PhD,** Associate Professor, Psychotherapy Program & Institute of Mental Health, Department of Psychiatry, The University of British Columbia, Vancouver, BC, Canada

Understanding Mechanisms of Change in Psychotherapies for Personality Disorders

Ueli **Kramer,**
Kenneth N. **Levy,**
and Shelley **McMain**

 AMERICAN PSYCHOLOGICAL ASSOCIATION

Published by
American Psychological Association
750 First Street, NE
Washington, DC 20002
https://www.apa.org

Order Department
https://www.apa.org/pubs/books
order@apa.org

Typeset in Charter and Interstate by Circle Graphics, Inc., Reisterstown, MD

Printer: Sheridan Books, Chelsea, MI
Cover Designer: Gwen J. Grafft, Minneapolis, MN

Library of Congress Cataloging-in-Publication Data

Names: Kramer, Ueli, author. | Levy, Kenneth N. (Kenneth Neil), 1963- author. | McMain, Shelley, author.
Title: Understanding mechanisms of change in psychotherapies for personality disorders / authored by Ueli Kramer, Kenneth N. Levy, and Shelley McMain.
Description: Washington, DC : American Psychological Association, [2024] | Includes bibliographical references and index.
Identifiers: LCCN 2023031496 (print) | LCCN 2023031497 (ebook) | ISBN 9781433836718 (paperback) | ISBN 9781433840951 (ebook)
Subjects: LCSH: Personality disorders. | Personality disorders--Treatment. | Psychotherapy--Methodology. | BISAC: PSYCHOLOGY / Psychopathology / Personality Disorders | PSYCHOLOGY / Psychotherapy / Counseling
Classification: LCC RC554 .K73 2024 (print) | LCC RC554 (ebook) | DDC 616.85/81--dc23/eng/20231103
LC record available at https://lccn.loc.gov/2023031496
LC ebook record available at https://lccn.loc.gov/2023031497

https://doi.org/10.1037/0000388-000

Printed in the United States of America

10 9 8 7 6 5 4 3 2 1

Contents

Understanding Mechanisms of **Change** in **Psychotherapies** for **Personality** Disorders

INTRODUCTION

Synthesizing Diverse Perspectives on Personality Disorders

We are aware, from our day-to-day clinical practice and years-long experience as psychotherapy researchers, that psychotherapy for patients with personality disorders can be both difficult and rewarding. As researchers, we are eager to improve the understanding of which treatments work best for this population and how these treatments work: We want to see more clinically informed psychotherapy research helping clinicians in their day-to-day work. As psychotherapists, we are humbly aware of the potential and the limitations of the therapy models we work with: We genuinely want to learn from what other treatment modalities have to offer. As human beings, we resonate with the inner and outer struggles of our patients, and we constantly attempt to give the best of us to help them.

At this juncture, we believe that what is needed for researchers and clinicians—somewhat boldly assuming that our own awareness and questions are relevant for others—is to take a step back and offer a consolidated synthesis of (a) what we know about how psychotherapies for personality disorders work and (b) what pressing clinically relevant questions the next generation of studies in psychotherapy should address. It is our pleasure to

https://doi.org/10.1037/0000388-001
Understanding Mechanisms of Change in Psychotherapies for Personality Disorders, by
U. Kramer, K. N. Levy, and S. McMain

invite you to meander with us toward a consolidated conceptualization of mechanisms of change in psychotherapies for personality disorders.

While we know that different psychotherapeutic treatments work, we know much less about how exactly they work. In this book, we examine psychotherapy for personality disorders with a focus on the mechanisms of change. Several prominent guidelines for the treatment of personality disorders, including those of the Society of Clinical Psychology's Committee on Science and Practice (https://div12.org/diagnosis/borderline-personality-disorder), the United Kingdom's National Institute for Health and Care Excellence (2009), the German Society for Psychiatry (Gaebel & Falkai, 2009), Australia's National Health and Medical Research Council (2012), the Swiss Association for Psychiatry and Psychotherapy (Euler et al., 2018), and the Netherlands Multidisciplinary Directive for Personality Disorders (Landelijke Stuurgroep Multidisciplinaire Richtlijnontwikkeling in de GGZ [Dutch Psychiatric Multidisciplinary Guideline Committee], 2008), all recommend psychotherapy as the first-line approach.

To date, no evidence demonstrates the superiority of one psychotherapy approach over another (see Cristea et al., 2017). Although theories of personality pathology and treatment are central to all psychotherapies, empirical evidence to explain how and why psychotherapy produces change is in the early stages. Given these limitations, evidence-informed practice is a process that requires an integration of the available relevant research and clinical wisdom. Diverse theories of psychotherapy and clinical perspectives exist, and these can result in points of tension and debate. The strengths of these points of tension or debate are that they pose opportunities to develop a broader perspective, build bridges between diverse perspectives, and advance our understanding of the complexity of psychotherapy. Finding syntheses between diverse methodologies, psychotherapy theories, and clinical practices will yield a richer and more precise understanding of the complexity of the psychotherapy. This endeavor is in line with the mission of the Society for the Exploration of Psychotherapy Integration (Goldfried et al., 2019).

This book seeks to establish practice-relevant knowledge by synthesizing the best available psychotherapy theories, empirical evidence, and clinical wisdom relevant to the treatment of personality disorders. We also seek to identify unanswered questions and maybe pose new ones that have the potential to inform psychotherapy research and practice for personality disorders in the future.

Within this focus on mechanisms of change, we highlight five specific domains of change anchored in a functional domain conception: emotion dysregulation, disturbed social interaction, identity problems, impulsivity, and cognitive disturbances. In each domain, we consider case formulations and clinical choice points arising from specific clinically challenging examples. These examples are based on our real-life clinical practice. Choice points in clinical practice are excellent ways to bring alive the transaction between research and practice. By doing so, we aim to articulate four levels of analysis: meta-analytic and randomized control trials, predictors and moderator research, findings from mechanisms of change and process research, and case formulation (see Chapter 1 for more details). In our presentation of the cases, we offer brief formulations of each case from our three perspectives, followed by an integrative formulation. Our discussions about clinical choice points culminate with clinical and research recommendations.

A SYNTHESIS OF KNOWLEDGE THROUGH EXPLORATORY DIALOGUES

For this book, in the absence of clear-cut data or an obvious path, we illustrate our clinical thinking regarding case formulations and clinical choice points, including our questions and doubts, via dialogues held between the three of us that were then transcribed and edited. These dialogues highlight both points of divergence and convergence among us and different theoretical orientations: plan analysis and the motive-oriented therapeutic relationship, in addition to clarification-oriented and emotion-focused therapies (represented by Ueli Kramer); transference-focused psychotherapy (represented by Kenneth Levy); and dialectical behavior therapy (represented by Shelley McMain).

Through our analysis of diverse theoretical perspectives and empirical evidence, we seek to attain a multilayered conception of synthesis of knowledge in science (Hassan & Will, 2006). General rules, as part of a discursive formation of the field of psychotherapy research, make it possible to study specific phenomena such as symptom change, human interaction, behavior, and emotion in psychotherapy. These objects of study may be differentiated into specific statements of concepts, such as psychotherapy outcome, the therapeutic relationship, and functional domains of personality. On the last layer of synthesis of scientific knowledge—or the "highest" in terms of abstraction—as outlined by Hassan and Will (2006), we may find the scientific theories, or models, themselves. On this layer of synthesis of scientific knowledge, among many others, the model of habituation to anxiogenic stimuli, the object relations theory, the model of vulnerability-stress, or the model of interpersonal hypersensitivity—all potentially relevant to explaining the treatment of personality disorders—may be cited. These theories contain a number of tenets (Hassan & Will, 2006) which may be operationalized and tested in empirical research in the interest of providing even more precise clinical recommendations.

We aim to be explicit about the tenets of our treatment models in our dialogues against the backdrop of clinical case material, highlight relevant empirical research, and consider different levels of analysis. We aim for a discourse marked by "a certain level of coherence, rigor, and stability" (Hassan & Will, 2006, p. 159). The last dialogue in this book (our discussion in Chapter 10) focuses on bringing these threads together by elaborating open questions for future research. In these dialogues aimed at consolidating knowledge, we must recognize that constructs have been developed and discussed within a specific scientific context (i.e., a theory or model with a history and specific tenets). Depending on the context, the meaning of a construct may slightly change. With regard to the origins of concepts, the current book will not delve into the details of the historical definition but aims to use a pragmatic and consensual approach.

The dialogues among us were held between 2019 and 2021, in person or conducted via Zoom. Of course, there was something spontaneous and unexpected in the process, almost like the spontaneity of a psychotherapy dialogue. This process allowed us to ground our thinking within a clinical context and build a more comprehensive understanding of the psychotherapy process. The majority of the dialogues started with a description of the patient and the specific clinical complaints associated with a functional domain-related personality pathology (for more on the functional domain, see Chapter 2). For each clinical case, we discuss our formulation and assessment and possible intervention strategies. In each case, we highlight choice points related to timing and focus that often arise in the course of therapy. We discuss our clinical formulations and interventions in light of empirical research and a consideration of different levels of analysis. We attempt to capitalize on and question underlying theoretical assumptions. We conclude each dialogue by synthesizing the key learnings from each case in terms of mechanisms of change in the treatment of personality disorders.

The kaleidoscope character of this book, the consolidated synthesis it provides, and the research perspectives it outlines take place in the context of relationships among us three. These relationships have developed over several years, and we express our gratitude for that. This book is not intended to be the final word on this subject; rather, it is meant to help further kick-start clinically informed science on mechanisms of change in psychotherapy. Through this endeavor, clinically relevant research questions will be formulated, and if they are put to an empirical test, we think they may yield results that inform the theory and practice of psychotherapy. As such, this book is mainly written for practicing psychotherapists and psychotherapists-in-training, in addition to psychotherapy researchers interested in developing clinically complex research questions. In addition, psychologists, psychiatrists, social workers, nurses, and other mental health practitioners may find this book helpful.

We aim for consolidated knowledge based on mechanisms of change in psychotherapy for personality disorders, and by doing so, we recognize the limitations of our method. First, a single clinical example cannot reflect all the diversity and complexity of a domain of functioning. We selected six relevant cases for the main chapters of this book out of a larger pool of cases to appropriately capture key features of specific domains of functioning. Other clinical examples may have yielded different content and choice points. For each case, we selected two to three clinical choice points that reflected opportunities for change. These choice points were selected because they were deemed highly relevant to a specific functional domain because they illustrated key challenges. We likely overlooked other important aspects of the cases, and this necessarily limits our conclusions. Finally, as in the practice of psychotherapy, our dialogues were marked by unpredictability, mutual responsiveness, and adjustments among the three of us along the way. We addressed these limitations by editing and summarizing and through a post-hoc analysis of our transcripts from each discussion. Again, the final result presented throughout the book is our read of the clinical material and the present state of the field. Our reflections are marked by an awareness of the huge potential of this kind of collaborative and integrative work for tailoring psychotherapy to the individual patient and for further research.

OVERVIEW OF THE BOOK'S STRUCTURE

The first two chapters provide a broad overview of the book's key themes. Chapter 1 reviews the importance of mechanisms of change when treating personality disorders, including how to determine the most optimal treatment for an individual patient. Chapter 2 reviews common mistaken claims about personality disorders, as well as the conceptualization of personality disorders within the five functional domains mentioned earlier: emotion dysregulation, disturbed social interaction, identity problems, impulsivity, and cognitive disturbances.

The next several chapters then review clinical guidelines for working with patients who have personality disorders. Chapter 3 answers frequently asked questions about how to approach the first session. It reviews common challenges associated with therapeutic collaboration and trust; criticisms of the therapist or the treatment; managing patients who engage in risky, self-harming, or suicidal behaviors; and developing a treatment framework. Chapters 4 to 8 then focus on each of the five functional domains, first providing brief reviews of empirical evidence when available before moving on to the case examples. Each chapter first provides a description of the patient and their presenting problems, followed by dialogues regarding case formulations and key choice points within therapy. These dialogues present our individual perspectives, followed by reviews of what they share and how they differ. Chapter 9 follows a similar format but focuses on challenges in the therapeutic relationship and how the therapist–patient alliance can help patients with personality disorders.

Chapter 10 concludes the book with a discussion that consolidates key takeaways from the previous dialogues and highlights future directions for research and practice.

ACKNOWLEDGMENTS

We would like to thank Susan Reynolds, Tyler Aune, David Becker, and their colleagues at the American Psychological Association for their support of this project and all anonymous reviewers whose feedback was most helpful to us. We thank the six clients with the pseudonyms Marcus, Janet, Leon, Arun, Irene, and Maria, who agreed that their material be used for this project and who have stimulated our thinking and dialogues on mechanisms of change in treatments of personality disorders.

1

THE IMPORTANCE OF DEVELOPING A FOCUS ON MECHANISMS OF CHANGE IN PSYCHOTHERAPY

As noted in the Introduction, this book focuses on mechanisms of change as a way to synthesize the strengths of various therapeutic approaches. This chapter goes into more detail about the empirical and theoretical basis for mechanisms of change as a way to understand and treat personality disorders. We first acknowledge the complexity of psychotherapy and the need for personalized psychotherapy; then, we discuss four levels of evidence when translating research results into practice using two case vignettes. This will help to understand the centrality of mechanisms of change in psychotherapy. We then discuss the theory's role in clinical practice and explain the methodology on the basis of dialogues in this book.

PERSONALIZING PSYCHOTHERAPY

In 1967, Gordon Paul famously asked the question, "What treatment, by whom, is most effective for this individual with that specific problem, and under which set of circumstances?" (p. 111). The art of implementing any treatment is customizing it to address the unique characteristics of each patient and context.

https://doi.org/10.1037/0000388-002
Understanding Mechanisms of Change in Psychotherapies for Personality Disorders, by U. Kramer, K. N. Levy, and S. McMain

The question of what works for whom, also known as aptitude-treatment interaction (Cronbach, 1957), acknowledges the importance of attending to individual differences in patients—differences that influence outcome as a function of treatment. This is what Sid Blatt and Irit Felsen (1993) referred to in the title of their article "Different Kinds of Folks May Need Different Kinds of Strokes." More generally, all psychotherapists ultimately endeavor to address the following question: "What is the best way to treat this person?" While this question seems simple, it is complex and far from straightforward.

Although many psychotherapies for personality disorders are effective, since Paul's (1967) famous query, there is a growing recognition that individuals respond differently to different treatments. For instance, even if we agree on how to define "efficacy," a therapy with a 75% efficacy rate—a limited index itself—means that one in four patients did not respond as fully as either they or we had hoped. Individuals who do not respond as fully as hoped for—sometimes called statistical "poor responders" or "nonresponders"—find themselves to be the collateral damage of allegedly evidence-based treatments. When one treatment fails to lead to change, individual patients are often left feeling uncertain about where to turn next and how best to proceed. They may blame themselves and not understand that the difficulty may lie in the limitations of the treatment or its application in their unique situation.

Although tailoring the psychotherapy treatment to the specifics of the patient, their difficulties, and the context has long been emphasized in the psychotherapy literature and can be seen clearly in Rogers's (1942) writings on person-centered therapy, the contemporary emphasis on personalizing psychotherapy has grown in tandem with the medical interest in genomic information (Hyman, 2010). Personalized treatment involves tailoring evidence-based treatment to the unique characteristics of each patient and clinical context. For example, a woman with a known genetic predisposition to breast cancer may receive more (and earlier in the process) in-depth screening than a woman without this genetic predisposition. This screening can improve the detection of illness and lead to early intervention and may result in a more effective treatment.

In the context of psychotherapy, knowing what works for whom requires an appreciation of the idiosyncratic characteristics of the individual. Clinicians need to consider clinically relevant and essential information when developing a treatment approach. For example, this often includes the identification of concurrent disorders. Individuals diagnosed with concurrent posttraumatic stress and borderline personality disorders may benefit from a psychotherapeutic approach that targets traumatic and borderline symptoms in an integrated fashion rather than a sequential approach. Failure to understand what is best for this unique patient can result in inadequate treatment, inappropriate care, and inefficient use of treatment resources. For example, an individual with borderline pathology and a learning disability may require additional support to make use of a skills training group. When an individual is engaged in a personalized plan of care, the patient, family, and health care system benefit. Ultimately, personalized approaches to psychotherapy hold promise for improving the efficiency and effectiveness of psychotherapy for the individual patient.

While personalizing psychotherapy appears to be a commonsense mission, appropriately individualizing treatment is not. Many biological, psychological, and social factors interact to determine individuals' response to therapy, and the on-the-ground complexity of psychotherapy makes individualized clinical decisions challenging. Translating empirical studies into clinical practice is complex and more of an artisanal process. Research findings do not always translate readily into clinical situations nor explain how to bring about change in the actual psychotherapy office. There needs to be a transactional flow of information between research and practice to facilitate the clinical relevance of research in the therapy practice. This may be because research essentially deals with general phenomena described in variables and psychotherapy deals with the idiosyncrasy of the case. Information gleaned from clinical practice should be informed by research questions such as "What is the best approach for an individual patient?" Research should also inform clinical practice so clinicians can address questions such as "What is the utility of this therapeutic strategy?" Clinicians, researchers, and consumers alike benefit from this intercommunication of research and practice.

CLINICAL VIGNETTES

To illustrate the complexity of clinical decision making relevant to individualize care, we consider two clinical cases.[1] We consider questions posed by these cases; elements of the patient's behavior, emotion and cognition, and environment will inform our decision making about the best approach for each patient.

The Case of Lara

Lara is a 22-year-old woman who presented to therapy after a breakup with her boyfriend, Carl. Since the breakup, she reported being unable to concentrate

---

[1]The case examples have been modified to disguise the patients' identities and protect their confidentiality.

at college. Her doctor recommended a prolonged medical leave for psychiatric reasons. Lara reported smoking marijuana regularly and engaging in heavy alcohol use involving frequent binge episodes since the age of 15. After her breakup with Carl, Lara increased her use of marijuana and alcohol. She also reportedly engaged in three episodes of self-harm behaviors involving superficial cuts to her forearms. Self-harm is a new behavior that alarmed her parents and teachers. During her first psychotherapy session, Lara felt unfairly treated by Carl, who left her for another woman. She described the breakup as particularly hurtful; it activated worries about her attractiveness and desirability to others. She noted that her trust in men was "shattered."

The Case of Theo

Theo is a 28-year-old man who presented to therapy after being asked to leave a PhD program in neuroscience. He presented as clinically depressed and reported sleep difficulties, suicidal ideation, angry outbursts triggered by minor difficulties, and a recent increase in problematic alcohol use. He reported that alcohol helped him because he "forgot the failure of my life." In response to a question about his future plans, he reported dreaming of becoming a renowned neuroscientist and successful researcher who unlocked the mysteries of the brain. In contrast to this dream, he had a lengthy history of failing to complete assignments throughout his graduate studies. He complained that his teachers were "unfair" and did not provide him with adequate support and guidance. He spoke with disdain and harsh words about his PhD advisor and boss. He acknowledged that it had always been difficult for him to accept guidance and interact with others in positions of authority. Notably, Theo's father is a prominent clerical figure in the Catholic church. Theo is gifted in mathematics and computer science. At the age of 18, Theo developed a new algorithm to disprove the existence of God. He reported that his proof failed, and he found it hard to recover from this failure experience. During the first session, Theo dismissively commented on an inquiry into his intimate life that he had no interest in women.

DETERMINING THE BEST TREATMENT APPROACH FOR A SPECIFIC PATIENT

There are multiple methods psychotherapists can use to select the most appropriate therapeutic approach for a patient. These include research-informed methods that involve four levels of analysis: a best-practices approach based on the patient's diagnosis, a heterogeneous approach that considers patient treatment responses, an approach focused on mechanisms of change, and a more detailed case formulation. Theory should also inform practice, particularly theories of mechanisms of change, which are core to this book's transtheoretical approach. Therapists must also consider the moment-by-moment responsive applications of these methods with an individual client, so we also discuss the importance of clinical choice points in this section.

Research-Informed Practice: Four Levels of Analysis

The selection of the optimal treatment approach for an individual patient can be guided by different levels of analysis. At a general level, many clinicians consider a patient's presenting symptoms and diagnoses and select a treatment approach suited to what is known about what works for the presenting problems. Best practices recommend selecting a treatment approach based on the best available relevant evidence. Best evidence usually comes from well-designed randomized controlled trials (RCTs) because they provide an estimate of treatment effects (Carey & Stiles, 2016; the first level of analysis).

The second level of analysis moves beyond using results of RCTs and concerns the heterogeneity of treatment responses. Selecting the appropriate treatment approach for an individual involves a consideration of the patient's environment and behavior relevant to their treatment response. Individual characteristics may have prescriptive (predictor variables) or prognostic (moderator variables) value. Predictor and moderator variables reveal information about an individual's response to treatment and allow for the selection of the most useful therapy approach. For example, the presence of posttraumatic stress disorder (PTSD) in individuals with borderline personality disorder (BPD) has been found in several studies (e.g., Boritz et al., 2016; Harned et al., 2008) to be associated with poor response, leading to adaptations of dialectical behavior therapy (DBT) for patients with comorbid BPD and PTSD.

The third level of analysis involves the selection of interventions that target the core processes and mechanisms associated with change in clinical outcomes. Mechanisms include the specific salutogenic processes taking place in the patient that contribute to change in some combination with the therapist intervention and the mechanisms driving specific psychopathological processes and their changes (Borkovec & Castonguay, 1998; Castonguay & Beutler, 2006a, 2006b; Castonguay et al., 2019; Goldfried, 1980; Goldfried & Wolfe, 1998; Kramer, 2018; Rosen & Davison, 2003). Selecting interventions from psychotherapies to target mechanisms of change and pathogenic processes can enhance the efficiency and effectiveness of treatment for the individual.

A fourth level of analysis entails understanding the individual's unique and subjective circumstances and tailoring treatment more precisely to the individual's experience. Many wise clinicians have long recognized that constructing a case formulation is an excellent way to make sense of the diverse pieces of relevant information about an individual. The importance of understanding the person to identify the best treatment approach dates back to Hippocrates, who said that it may be more important to know what sort of person has a disease than to know what sort of disease a person has.

Psychotherapy is complex, and each of these four levels of analysis addresses a different perspective and clinically relevant issue. The synthesis of knowledge gained through these multiple levels of analysis can increase our understanding of how to optimize psychotherapy for the individual patient within context. In the next section, these levels of analysis are applied to the cases of Lara and Theo.

Level 1: General Treatment Approach for Personality Disorders

The first level of analysis involves an assessment of the patient's symptoms and diagnoses and the selection of a suitable treatment that is relevant to the patient's diagnostic profile. An emphasis on the findings of RCTs and meta-analytic studies is used to identify the most suitable treatment. Will a suitable treatment for Lara or Theo be informed by the treatment recommendations based on RCTs? What diagnosis best describes the symptoms of Lara and Theo? Lara and Theo both meet the criteria for BPD. Lara exhibits interpersonal difficulties, episodes of self-harm, frequent impulsive behaviors, and difficulty with emotional control. Theo displays identity problems, transient difficulties with reality testing, and emotional difficulties.

The results of several RCTs and meta-analyses indicate that several therapeutic approaches are effective for patients with personality disorders. Over the past 30 years, outcome research has largely focused on evaluating the treatment of BPD (Cristea et al., 2017; Storebø et al., 2020) and demonstrated positive effects of several approaches across a broad range of outcomes. The effects of psychotherapy for other personality disorders are less clear, though several strong outcome studies exist (Budge et al., 2013).

Notwithstanding this rather good news, there are limitations to the empirical support for BPD-specific psychotherapies that limit the relevance of research findings. To date, most RCTs have compared active treatments with treatment-as-usual conditions. Few direct comparisons exist between active treatments. Consequently, there is limited evidence to address which approach works best for whom.

A few head-to-head trials evaluated the efficacy of one approach over an alternative treatment. A dismantling study by Linehan et al. (2015)

evaluated the effectiveness of standard DBT compared with individual therapy and with skills training (offered in group settings) alone and found no overall difference in the three conditions on the primary outcome, suicide attempts. Conditions that included skills training were superior to individual therapy alone on some secondary outcomes, including self-harm. McMain and colleagues (2009, 2012) compared the clinical effectiveness of DBT with general psychiatric management (GPM) and a psychodynamic approach for the treatment of self-harming individuals diagnosed with BPD. Findings indicated no between-condition differences on any outcomes at the end of the 1-year treatment and 36-month follow-up. A study by Clarkin, Levy, et al. (2007) comparing transference-focused psychotherapy (TFP), DBT, and a psychodynamic supportive therapy found that all three treatments were effective in reducing anxiety and depression and improving global and social adjustment. In terms of differences between conditions, TFP showed superiority in reducing aggression compared with DBT, and supportive therapy was less effective than TFP and DBT for suicidal and anger outcomes. Finally, Bateman and Fonagy (2009) compared mentalization-based therapy with a structured clinical management and found that both treatments improved core symptoms of BPD. What has become clear is that few substantial differences between active treatments exist.

Several meta-analytic studies (e.g., Storebø et al., 2020) similarly show no evidence for the superiority of one psychotherapeutic approach over another for BPD, leading many to conclude what some researchers call the dodo bird verdict for the treatment of this disorder: All have won, and everyone must have prizes! While this is encouraging news, there are limitations to the existing research, and it is premature to conclude that all therapies produce the same outcomes. RCTs report group effects; these necessarily over- or underestimate the effect for an individual, who will not, for example, experience a 75% improvement from a treatment with 75% efficacy but rather fall into either the 75% who improve or the 25% who do not. It may be that some patients respond better to a specific model or format of therapy.

The long-term effects of psychotherapy are rarely assessed, and the long-term durability of treatment effects is unknown. Given what we know about the decades-long evolution of BPD as a disorder within individuals (Gunderson et al., 2011; Zanarini, 2019), understanding the durability of treatment effects is important. Further, there is also limited evidence to guide decisions about the appropriate dosage of psychotherapy. In a Cochrane meta-analysis (Storebø et al., 2020), almost half (48%) of the studies included treatments that were shorter than 6 months. These studies demonstrate that strong and clinically reliable changes can be achieved in shorter durations of treatment. At the same time, the durability of the treatment effects of short-term therapies compared with longer term therapy is unknown, but clinical experience and observational data tend to suggest that this may be the case.

Our first level of analysis provides hopeful information about the efficacy of psychotherapy for personality disorders. The knowledge that a treatment is effective may be sufficient for some clinicians. However, most clinicians recognize that, in practice, it is not always possible to implement an evidence-based treatment with a high level of integrity. Furthermore, even if the treatment is delivered with a high level of integrity, it may be insufficient for an individual patient.

The effect of psychotherapy for people with personality disorders may be akin to the effect of taking an aspirin to tackle a headache: Facing symptoms (the headache), the person takes the correct dose of aspirin, and subsequently, the symptom (the headache) disappears. From a strictly logical viewpoint, the patient does not need to question why and how the aspirin brought about the change in headache. However, what if the headache does not go away after taking the correct dose of aspirin? In this situation, when the treatment does not work, it is important for the patient to consider additional information, such as what to do when the correct dose is insufficient. Knowledge about nonresponders is usually overlooked in RCTs and understanding factors that contributed to poor or no response will improve the effectiveness of therapy for all.

In the case of Lara and Theo, knowing that each patient meets the diagnostic criteria for BPD suggests a course of action different from the recommended treatment for other disorders, such as obsessive-compulsive disorder or psychotic disorder. While diagnostic information is valuable for the clinician, it is not sufficient.

It is not known whether Lara or Theo would respond better to one therapy approach or format over another. First, Lara and Theo both meet the criteria for three to four other mental health disorders. For example, Lara meets the criteria for a substance use disorder, and it is not clear whether Lara's substance abuse should be prioritized over other disorders. Second, in both cases, the patients manifest BPD symptoms differently. For example, in Theo's case, it is not clear if the therapist should prioritize deeper psychic issues such as self-identity or prioritize his symptoms and suicidality. BPD, in general, is a heterogeneous disorder associated with high rates of concurrent disorders. Consequently, clinicians need to make a nuanced assessment of the patient's characteristics and environment to make a clinical decision about the best treatment approach. To date, research has not resulted in compelling evidence about how to apply a personalized approach.

Level 2: Predictors and Moderators of Treatment Response

Research on predictors and moderators of psychotherapy outcomes can help advance the field of personalized treatment for personality disorders. Predictors and moderators facilitate the identification of people who may be at risk for poor outcomes and could benefit from different interventions. Predictor variables are factors that foreshadow ("predict") response to treatment and can help identify people who are at risk for poor outcomes. For example, specific genes for breast cancer can predict response to treatment. Taken as a whole, predictor variables provide clues about which treatments need to be tailored to specific subgroups of patients and can enable more helpful treatment. In contrast, moderator variables provide prescriptive information on whether a patient will do better with one treatment over another. For example, a patient with a specific breast cancer gene who is otherwise healthy may be at risk for poor outcomes with one form of chemotherapy compared with another.

For patients with BPD, such as Theo and Lara, research into which approach is most promising for them and how they will respond is still limited. In a meta-analysis of predictor studies (Barnicot et al., 2012), among the host of variables examined, only two variables significantly predicted treatment success in BPD: high intensity of symptoms at pretreatment and a good therapeutic alliance. Such information about which variables predict outcomes is valuable in guiding clinical decision making.

A handful of studies have examined moderators of treatment outcomes in samples of patients treated for personality disorders. Preliminary evidence indicates that specific factors, such as level of psychopathology, moderate the response to psychotherapy outcomes for BPD. For example, a study by Gullestad et al. (2013) involved a mixed sample of patients with personality disorders randomized to outpatient therapy or a day treatment program. The authors found that those with low pretreatment mentalization responded better to outpatient treatment than to the comparator treatment. The researchers speculated that the intensive day treatment program may have been inferior for patients with lower mentalization because the program required the navigation of multiple relationships and may have overstimulated the patients' attachment systems. A single variable is unlikely to have sufficient clinical utility, and with the advancement of more sophisticated statistical modeling, it is possible to examine multiple moderators of treatment response.

A study by Keefe et al. (2020) examined multiple moderators of treatment response using the personalized advantage index (PAI) methodology. This method examines moderators on the individual patient level and is particularly well suited to identifying the best therapy approach for a particular patient profile. A combination of specific patient characteristics was found to moderate response to 1 year of DBT over GPM for BPD. Whereas the original RCT comparing DBT with GPM revealed no difference on any outcomes at 12, 24, and 36 months (McMain et al., 2009, 2012), the PAI methodology revealed that DBT performed best with patients who were more dependent, more psychosocially impaired, and who exhibited higher levels of childhood trauma. In contrast, GPM was superior for patients who were symptomatically complex and had higher general symptoms and borderline symptoms. While this information is relevant, we lack studies to draw more firm conclusions.

Applied to our two cases, we expect that Lara and Theo have a fairly good chance of treatment success. They both have a high level of symptoms, and this predicts a good outcome. The course of treatment may need to be adapted as new information emerges, such as the disclosure of a childhood history of trauma. In addition, it will be important to monitor the therapeutic alliance, including the degree of collaboration, agreement on tasks and goals, and the bond between patient and therapist.

Research evidence on predictors and moderators does not readily translate to clinical practice. Pretreatment characteristics may be useful in predicting how patients respond to treatment; however, how to intervene with a patient who is expected to have a poor response remains unclear. It seems rash to deny a patient a course of treatment simply on the basis of the presence of a characteristic that predicts a poor response. It seems more appropriate to consider how to strengthen the treatment. It is well known that treatment outcomes are determined by multiple factors, some unknown, and considering one factor is too simplistic.

Level 3: Principles, Processes, and Mechanisms of Change

Research on mechanisms of change addresses the question of how psychotherapy works and advances our understanding of how to personalize therapy. According to Kazdin (2009), a mechanism of change is a variable that produces or statistically explains the outcome of psychotherapy. It is a type of *changing variable*—a variable that enacts, enables, or is otherwise functionally responsible for the change observed. This changing variable, to properly be considered a mechanism of change, must show systematic association with the outcome and a direct effect on the change in symptoms subsequent to treatment outcome. Mechanisms of change must be consistent with existing clinical theories of psychotherapy and psychopathology, be the subject of systematic study across research programs, and be validated in experimental research. In applying such a rigorous definition, no variable has so far made the cut to be categorized as a valid mechanism of change in psychotherapy for personality disorders. This does not mean that there is no research in the field or that psychotherapies lack theories on putative mechanisms of change but rather the research is incomplete and deserves more systematic attention. We understand that our work untangles pathways to change by summarizing the empirical evidence of mechanisms of change and intertwining this information with clinical wisdom. We hope to contribute to knowledge on the practice of psychotherapy for personality disorders by identifying practical intermediate outcomes as patients progress through treatment. At this juncture, we are left with many questions about how to bring about change, and we hope that these questions will stimulate future research.

The psychotherapy research field is moving beyond an exclusive focus on evidence-based treatment to an increased emphasis on the personalization of therapy. Understanding the specific mechanisms and processes that underlie change is vital to knowing how and why specific variables produce treatment outcomes. In this way, mechanisms of change research is closely interrelated to the aim of personalized treatment. Doss (2004) differentiated between therapist interventions, processes of change, and mechanisms of change: Processes of change take place as a response to therapist interventions in the psychotherapy hour, whereas mechanisms of change involve targeted functions that are changing in the patient, both in session and in daily life as a result of psychotherapy. For example, certain therapy interventions may elicit in-session emotional processes that strengthen the image the person has of themself (the latter is the targeted mechanism responsible for outcome). We argue that, after all, patients engage in therapy to make changes in their life, not simply to change in the therapy hour, though change in the therapy hour may be key to changes outside of therapy.

Investigating mechanisms of change in treatment involves asking questions about the steps that lead the patient toward improvement over the course of therapy. Clinical interest in mechanisms can play out as an interest in intermediate treatment goalposts linked to mechanisms of change. But despite the significance of understanding mechanisms of change in psychotherapy, there is a dearth of knowledge when it comes to identifying intermediate treatment goals and how they relate to the patient's short- and long-term goals in treatment (Cuijpers, 2019). Different therapy approaches define intermediate objectives—or corollary proposed mechanisms of change—in different ways, seldom acknowledging possible overlaps, similarities, and differences.

One approach to synthesize different approaches involves the notion of principles of change. According to an important book by Castonguay and Beutler (2006b), *Principles of Therapeutic Change That Work*, principles of change are relevant to mechanisms of change but do not completely overlap. Castonguay and Beutler identified four perspectives on principles of change: participant (patients and therapists), relationship between participants, technical correlates of these perspectives, and an integrative conception of them. These four contributions are examined within categories of specific psychological difficulties (among them, personality disorders). Another contribution to the notion of principles of change is the five factors of change in the theory by Grawe (1998), an example of theoretical integration in psychotherapy. According to Grawe, all psychotherapies may function because of the operation of five factors that interact with each other and can be explicitly fostered by the therapist: clarification of motivation, coping with problems or mastery, processual activation of problems, resource activation, and the therapeutic relationship.

Principles of change and mechanisms of change are similar but are not the same (Goldfried, 1980, 2019). Principles of change are conceptualized at a mid-level of abstraction that avoids the treatment approach–specific language of psychotherapy techniques and the generic and often clinically too-abstract constructs of possible kernels of change that happen in the patient irrespective of the treatment approach. Mechanisms of change, however, are concepts that link an approach-specific conceptualization and theorization, treatment tasks, and techniques with observable patient processes. Mechanisms of change account for the patient's processes of change in interaction with therapist interventions, strategies, and conceptualizations. As such, mechanisms of change may represent, to some extent, an operationalization of more mid-level abstractions (i.e., principles of change) and may be observed in the process of psychotherapy research and practice. This explains the great potential of mechanisms of change for both psychotherapy research and practice.

General knowledge that a psychotherapy approach can alleviate symptoms is helpful; however, information about mechanisms of change can inform decisions about how to optimize the active ingredients of therapy. Clarifying intermediate outcomes and focusing on how to adapt therapy to address the needs of individual patients in a step-by-step responsive fashion holds the promise of improving outcomes. Though general knowledge about the best approach for BPD is a starting point, the unique clinical characteristics of Lara and Theo raise questions about how to optimize therapy for these patients and their unique characteristics. In subsequent chapters of this book, we explore how therapy can be targeted to address specific problems as distinct functional domains. This targeted methodology moves us beyond our earlier levels of analysis (i.e., general treatment approach) into a more individualized analysis of the patient and a consideration of the core principles, processes, and mechanisms of change explaining treatment response. Individualization of therapy is interlinked with therapeutic change components because the active ingredients of treatment can vary according to the unique circumstances of the person, disorder, comorbidity, and context.

What are the implications of understanding these theorized mechanisms of change for the treatment of Lara and Theo? DBT may address Lara's emotional dysregulation, which figures centrally in her presentation. Validation, dialectical strategies, and skills training are strategies that could be used to help her modulate her emotions and interrupt impulsive behaviors (e.g., substance use and self-harm behavior). Theo presents with pronounced identity problems, including concerns about professional identity, sexual identity, and a fragile sense of self, and he may benefit more from the explicit focus of TFP on identity. In other words, therapists could identify the patient's core symptoms and match the model best suited to address specific mechanisms.

In the next section, we briefly review a few studies that exemplify the potential benefits of gleaning clinical direction from research on mechanisms and processes of change. These studies are part of a larger and accumulating body of research that aims to support the putative mechanisms of change proposed in numerous psychotherapies and that is often borne out by clinical observation.

The first study by Levy et al. (2006) focused on the role of changes in reflective functioning, an operationalization of the concept of mentalization, in a sample of patients diagnosed with BPD who were enrolled in TFP, DBT, or supportive therapy. Results revealed that an increase in reflective functioning was observed only in TFP patients, who engaged in different, potentially more elaborate, and complex ways of reflecting on others in the course of adult attachment interviews. Patients in DBT and supportive therapy did not exhibit this increased reflective functioning. TFP was also associated with changed attachment patterns indicative of a more stable attachment formation, which was observed less in the other two conditions. According to psychodynamic theory, these changed mentalization and attachment patterns reflect a deeper change in how patients maintain early representations and apply them to present relationships. And insofar as a patient's recovery needs to involve stabilized attachment patterns, the patient may require a treatment whose mechanism of change involves attachment. Achieving higher reflective functioning in the adult attachment interview could be a principle of change reflecting the putative mechanism of change, which is stabilized attachment patterns. Given an awareness of what mechanisms constitute the active ingredients of the treatment, a provider can identify an ideal candidate for TFP according to whether their specific challenges align with those ingredients underlying TFP success. In this way, a grasp of the research literature on mechanisms of change can meaningfully inform clinical decision making. We can also see how research-informed decision making enables a more individualized and personalized approach to treatment.

The second study is by McMain et al. (2013), focusing on the role of improvements in affect balance in DBT and good psychiatric management. The researchers found that even after controlling for the contribution of the therapeutic alliance, improvements in affect balance were significantly associated with decreased psychiatric symptom distress and interpersonal problems. The results of this study suggest that one of the mechanisms through which DBT and alternative treatments of BPD may effectively reduce symptom distress and interpersonal problems is greater symmetry of positive and negative affect. We can keep this putative mechanism of change in mind when considering the clinical presentation of patients, such that DBT surfaces as a strong contender for the treatment of patients who display particular affect distress.

The third study, by Kramer et al. (2017), focused on the decrease in behavioral coping in BPD (i.e., the reduction of impulsive and other behavioral ways of dealing with a stressor). A decrease in behavioral coping early in psychiatric treatment arose as a potential statistical mediator of the effects of individualized case formulation (to be discussed further under Level 4). The researchers found that for patients who received treatment with a motive-oriented therapeutic relationship, the symptom reduction observed between Sessions 5 and 10 was indeed mediated by a reduction of behavioral coping observed between Sessions 1 and 5. What that may mean for clinicians is that early reduction of behavioral coping may indicate that the psychiatric treatment is "on track" and "good enough," while for patients who do not show this type of early change, it may be advisable for the therapist to focus explicitly on these behavioral problems (e.g., by adding a DBT intervention).

So far, we know that the treatment for Lara and Theo may be multifaceted and vary according to individual differences and the therapist's interpretation of them. The next steps in selecting the best treatment may depend on earlier decisions made by the patient and the therapist. Depending on the availability of a specific evidence-based treatment in a particular health care context, the therapist's allegiance to a specific model, and the patient's explicit demand for a specific treatment based on preexisting information and other contextual factors, one or the other available options may be taken. The chosen focus may adaptively and dynamically change as a function of the completion (vs. noncompletion) of intermediate treatment objectives and outcomes. Several roads may lead to Rome, and it is the norm for those roads to wind and even abruptly change direction in ways that both challenge and inspire the therapist who makes clinically rooted and research-informed decisions along the way.

Much of the research we have described offers specific guidance to the therapist learning how to navigate those roads. The therapist now knows that, through TFP, change in attachment patterns is possible through specific psychodynamic work linking early representations to the current affective and relationship experience, through using what is happening in the transference, and through undoing some of the negative and unhelpful interaction patterns from the past. The therapist now knows that, as seen in DBT and GPM, change in emotional and cognitive expression are feasible, and focusing on establishing balance may be a helpful treatment target. And the therapist now knows that early in treatment, based on a structured case formulation of the patient's problems, the focus on reducing the behavioral ways of coping is a highly promising initial treatment target.

What remains unanswered about the best treatment for Lara and Theo is how to tailor the information from these studies and others to the individual patient. The final stretch of our journey that brings us full circle between practice and research concerns case formulation.

Level 4: Case Formulation
Several psychotherapies could be helpful for Lara and Theo. Common factors (e.g., therapeutic alliance and goal setting) and differences across these models and change related to each model are associated with specific mechanisms of action, and thus the model should be chosen for suitability to the patient's challenges and therapeutic needs. Yet, despite this knowledge, there is a gap in knowing how to integrate empirical evidence with the unique aspects of a case. Personal characteristics and environmental factors vary from individual to individual and require fine-grained decisions that cannot be captured by information on predictor and moderator variables and the general mechanisms of change.

Case formulation is a tool assumed to be indispensable to psychotherapy because it ties generic knowledge to the features of each patient. A case formulation is used to organize specific information about a patient, increase understanding and empathy for the patient's situation, and inform a treatment plan and intervention. In the development of a case formulation, idiosyncratic mechanisms of change that may define an individual patient's recovery can emerge.

Kramer (2019) presented ideas from major theoretical models and illustrated key features of case formulation in the treatment of personality disorders and how it informs treatment planning (Kramer, 2019). While case formulation is considered an essential skill in most schools of therapy, the evidence for treatment guided by a case formulation is mixed. Some research shows that therapy guided by a structured case formulation is associated with a stronger treatment effect than therapy conducted without a formal case formulation. For example, one randomized controlled trial of BPD treatment found that treatment guided by a structured case formulation was associated with superior reductions in general symptoms (Kramer et al., 2014); however, there was no added benefit to diminishing borderline symptoms in this study. These effects were comparable to a study on the additional effect of case formulation on outcome in the treatment of bulimia (Ghaderi, 2006). Other research found that therapy augmented by a structured case formulation was not associated with any additional benefits (Emmelkamp et al., 1994). One study on exposure for the treatment of anxiety disorders found that the use of a case formulation was associated with poor effects when compared with a manual-based approach (Schulte et al., 1992), although one must note that the case formulations made in this early study missed several elements necessary from a contemporary perspective. Kramer (2020) discussed methodological challenges that make this type of research difficult but not impossible to implement.

While acknowledging the open questions and limitations regarding the effective utility of a case formulation, we recognize that it guides the personalization of treatment, helps to develop an understanding of individual differences, and increases the chances of better outcomes. Taken alone without earlier levels of analysis, there is no evidence that it is a sufficient tool. But the art of treatment is using multiple tools to supplement each level's shortcomings while taking advantage of skills that may otherwise be too quickly dismissed. In subsequent sections of this book, we explore how case formulation can be used in tandem with other reasoning to advance stronger clinical decision making.

How Does a Case Formulation Apply to Lara and Theo?

In the case of Lara, a DBT therapist may engage the patient in a detailed chain analysis to understand the function of the behavior. In Lara's case, self-harm is typically triggered by perceived rejection from others, such as the breakup with Carl. A trigger such as rejection may activate underlying feelings of loneliness and Lara's negative self-view that she is incapable of functioning. By assessing the function of the patient's self-harm behavior, the therapist and patient can focus on treating the essence of the problem— the patient's intolerance of being alone and her self-criticism. Solutions may include increasing the patient's mindfulness of her feelings of loneliness and practicing exposure to emotions to modify aversive emotions.

In Theo's case, from an object-relational perspective such as that used in TFP, we may understand that his sense of self oscillates between two positions: (a) a sense of self as a math and computer genius in the eyes of others and (b) a sense of self as a complete failure who feels ashamed of himself. This differentiated view then offers a perspective of how Theo views himself—which will be used in insight-enhancing treatment—and also offers a perspective on how the separated views of himself may be integrated into a more coherent representation of the self.

These case formulations can develop a coherent framework for understanding the patient's situation at a finer grain of detail than any broader form of analysis (see also Caspar et al., 2010). But even when a case formulation is developed flawlessly in one model or approach, there are invariably factors that are overlooked if broader levels of analysis, such as those described in earlier sections, are not simultaneously considered. Each therapy model differs in terms of information that it considers important and relevant, and before reaching a case formulation on one particular model, earlier levels of analysis can point the therapist toward the right framework. Likewise, one case formulation method is steeped in a particular theory; therefore, increasing the therapist's knowledge of alternative formulation methods and their application will likely lead to more complete and comprehensive formulations.

How do these levels of analysis inform treatment decision making in the cases of Lara and Theo? Critical appraisal of information from our four levels of analysis is central to more informed clinical decision making. Therapists need to consider the patient in light of their characteristics and how the available evidence and knowledge can meaningfully inform treatment. Additional research in each area of diagnosis-related studies, predictors and moderators, mechanisms of change, and improved case formulation will help to advance both theoretical and applied knowledge and improve our ability to increase the precision in the process of personalization of therapy for patients like Lara and Theo.

THEORY-INFORMED PRACTICE

Basing clinical decisions only on empirical evidence is insufficient because the research literature is incomplete, and the gaps in scientific knowledge cannot be ignored. Any wise practitioner recognizes that it is reasonable to incorporate other forms of knowledge, including clinical wisdom and theoretical knowledge, to inform decisions on the best treatment for a specific patient. As a Yale University student stated in 1882, "In theory there is no difference between theory and practice, while in practice there is" (Brewster, p. 202). In this next section, we consider different theories of psychotherapy and how theory informs our third level of analysis—mechanisms of change.

A central goal of this book is to highlight the benefits of integrating multiple and diverse theoretical perspectives. Toward this goal, we begin by examining how distinct theories conceptualize mechanisms of change. Mechanisms of change play a significant role in translating theory into clinical practice. While these mechanisms are one of other relevant levels of analysis, we consider them especially important and relevant to linking underlying theory to clinical assessment and intervention.

Theories of Mechanisms of Change

Psychotherapy theories have been developed to explain psychopathology but differ in terms of the key theorized mechanisms responsible for change (Prochaska & Norcross, 2014). We contrast and synthesize the different theoretical positions of the diverse perspectives we outline in this book. Briefly, we outline the key theorized mechanisms responsible for change in specific therapy approaches.

From a DBT perspective, change in outcomes occurs directly or indirectly through the enhancement of emotion-regulation capacities (Linehan, 1993). In their conceptualization of mentalization-based therapy, Fonagy and Bateman (2006) proposed that "the enhancement of mentalization and the reduction of the predominance of non-mentalising modes of experiencing internal reality represent the path to cure" (p. 414). From a TFP perspective, it is necessary to modify the patient's mental representations (i.e., perceptions) of self and others to effect change in symptoms. From a plan analysis and motive-oriented therapeutic relationship perspective, change in outcomes arises through the conditions associated with corrective emotional experiences in the therapy relationship, which foster further changes in therapy (Caspar, 2019, 2022). In cognitive behavior therapy, modifying core dysfunctional beliefs is necessary to produce change (Davidson et al., 2006). In schema therapy (Young et al., 2003), recovery involves the transformation of maladaptive schema modes, including the reduction of maladaptive schemas and the strengthening of adaptive schemas. From the perspective of good psychiatric management, to effect change, it is necessary to raise patients' awareness of their interpersonal hypersensitivity (Gunderson & Links, 2014). From a clarification-oriented psychotherapy perspective, to effect change, it is necessary to increase insight by activating the patient's representation of self and others in the here-and-now interpersonal domain (Sachse, 2020). In emotion-focused therapy, change in outcomes occurs through the transformation of maladaptive emotions into adaptive emotional processing (Greenberg, 2019).

The juxtaposition of theorized mechanisms raises questions about these theorized constructs. Some of the described theorized processes represent unique information, while some describe similar and largely overlapping processes, and it is a matter of language what a specific mechanism is called. It is possible that treatments work for treatment-specific reasons; however, common factors likely account for changes in outcomes. Little research has been devoted to understanding whether specific therapies may work for reasons other than those theorized, although such research may be highly welcome for an integrative understanding of mechanisms of change (for an exception, see the analysis of defense mechanisms as mechanisms of change in DBT; Euler et al., 2019). As discussed, confirming any of these theoretical assumptions, while important, may likely be insufficient for improving outcomes. Using a more idiographic approach, targeting the purported specific mechanisms of the individual patient may optimize treatment outcomes.

The Person of the Psychotherapist Within Mechanisms of Change

The person of the therapist is a central factor relevant to treatment outcomes: It refers to the personal and professional qualities of the therapist in the therapeutic process, in addition to the skills the person of the therapist masters in facing clinical challenges. Although the qualities of a therapist are a potent element of change in psychotherapy, this topic has received little attention in the research literature until recently. Across psychotherapy research studies, a consistent finding is that not all therapists are equally effective in treating patients (Castonguay & Hill, 2017). The variability between patient outcomes across therapists is as high as 2:1, meaning that, with some exceptions, some therapists in the community produce outcomes twice as good as those of less-effective therapists.

While understanding therapist effects is in its infancy from a research perspective (Castonguay & Hill, 2017), it is important to describe helpful features of particularly effective psychotherapists (and unhelpful features of others). In treating patients with personality disorders, Fernandez-Alvarez et al. (2006) observed that effective therapists have the following characteristics: an open-minded and creative attitude, a flexible therapeutic approach, comfort with emotionally intense interactions, tolerance and mindfulness of their own emotions (including negative feelings toward the patient and the therapeutic process), and patience. It is reasonable to assume that therapists who receive sufficient training in evidence-based treatment(s), accompanied by intense case supervision, are best equipped to treat patients with personality disorders effectively.

WORKING IN PSYCHOTHERAPY USING CHOICE POINTS

Therapists are faced with numerous choice points in psychotherapy. Clinical choice points—decision points about the therapist's next move—may arise at the macro level, such as decisions about the general treatment approach (our Level 1), and may arise at micro levels, such as when making decisions about what to do in a challenging moment in therapy (our Level 3).

Psychotherapy process researchers have studied moment-by-moment changes in the tasks characterizing in-session "events" (Rice & Greenberg, 1984). The detailed, microscopic analysis of such events has contributed to the knowledge of how specific events unfold, including patient markers and how they shift, evolve, and eventually resolve and what the therapist does to navigate these challenges. For example, challenging moments studied by research, which become highly relevant choice points for clinical intervention and especially for patients with personality disorders, include the working through of self-critical splits (Greenberg, 1984; Kramer, Blanco Machinea, et al., 2023) and the negotiation of a rupture in the therapeutic alliance (Muran & Eubanks, 2020). For our purpose, such in-session events may become choice points of intervention in that they (a) are possibly linked to a specific clinical feature (i.e., a functional domain linked to a personality disorder; see Chapter 2) and (b) represent an opportunity for change in the particular moment. Taken together (a and b), choice points become research-based and clinically relevant moments of preferential intervention by a therapist focusing on mechanisms of change, helping the patient move toward resolution. The identification of choice points may therefore be relevant for (a) the practitioner (i.e., they will learn what can be done in response to a specific clinical challenge) and (b) the researcher (i.e., they will learn how to implement an assessment of potential mechanisms of change that is event related and clinically relevant).

Choice points involve integrating research with clinical expertise and individual characteristics of the therapist and patient. Good clinical judgment involves not only an assessment of the facts of the situation but also the ability to combine relevant knowledge, clinical expertise, and an individualized case formulation. It requires continuous monitoring of the therapy process to identify what works and what is less helpful.

CONCLUSIONS

To summarize, diverse perspectives and a consolidated synthesis of ideas from different therapy models is needed in psychotherapy for personality disorders. A synthesis of diverse perspectives has the potential to advance the field and knowledge on how to personalize psychotherapy. Not all patients respond to all treatments, and diverse knowledge may expand clinicians' understanding of how to work with individual patients and ultimately enhance the effectiveness of psychotherapy. Research on mechanisms of change in psychotherapies is a promising way to foster a common language, along with conceptual clarity, between researchers and clinicians from different theoretical orientations.

In addition to the four pathways to psychotherapy integration, including theoretical integration, technical eclecticism, assimilative integration, and integration via common factors (see also Norcross & Goldfried, 2019), a focus on mechanisms of psychotherapy is another avenue for integration across diverse approaches. Understanding mechanisms of change may help a therapist know how to foster specific processes of change, leading to a more personalized psychotherapeutic approach. Focusing on mechanisms of change in treatments for personality disorders may be especially fruitful when different theoretical perspectives are considered, and a synthesis of perspectives informs clinical practice. A discussion about divergent and convergent threads is required to move toward a consolidation of knowledge.

2 PERSONALITY DISORDERS

A Conceptualization in Functional Domains

In this chapter, we discuss different conceptualizations of personality disorders, examine current and past controversies in the field, and propose a functional domain conceptualization of personality disorder and personality pathology. Functional domains, as defined here, are not the only a useful way to conceptualize personality disorders, but we believe they provide a useful framework.

Our goal is to provide a basis for integrating current theory and research to help clinicians navigate complex and confusing clinical material while working with patients who present with personality pathology. We use a functional domain framework throughout this book and discuss the features of identified functional domains (e.g., emotional dysregulation, problematic social interaction) that are then illustrated through clinical examples to guide interventions. Our approach integrates diverse theoretical models, empirical evidence, and case formulations.

https://doi.org/10.1037/0000388-003
Understanding Mechanisms of Change in Psychotherapies for Personality Disorders, by
U. Kramer, K. N. Levy, and S. McMain

CONCEPTUALIZATION OF PERSONALITY DISORDERS

In the 19th and 20th centuries, several conceptual lenses of personality disorders were put forth to conceptualize personality pathology. For example, Kraepelin (1907), Bleuler (1911), and Kretschmer (1925) described personality types such as asthenic, autistic, schizoid, and cyclothymic (or cycloid) and viewed them as premorbid personalities to schizophrenic and manic-depressive disorders. Contrasting with modern views of personality disorders, they were seen as akin to temperaments and considered a form of psychotic experience. In contrast, Karl Jaspers (1923/1963) viewed personality difficulties as developing independently from medically defined symptoms and originating from an individual's premorbid personality structure and functioning. Later, Stern (1938), who was often credited with coining the term borderline personality, described several features of what we now regard as borderline personality disorder (BPD). This included devaluation and idealization of the therapist and a difficulty controlling emotions, leading to "psychic bleeding." He observed the strong countertransferential reactions evoked in clinicians in response to these patients. From a psychoanalytic perspective, Stern (1938) viewed personality disorders as stemming from an individual's personality or character rather than a condition of insanity or a true medical condition such as psychosis. Deutsch (1942) and Kernberg (1968) were responsible for transforming conceptualizations of personality disorders. Despite their efforts, personality disorder—especially BPD—was long considered a form of schizophrenia, as evidenced by its inclusion in the *Diagnostic and Statistical Manual of Mental Disorders* (2nd ed.; *DSM-II*; American Psychiatric Association, 1968) under the moniker of *latent schizophrenia*.

Later, psychoanalysts began to differentiate between types of personality disorders, as evidenced by their descriptions of patients with narcissistic features. Kernberg (1967, 1970, 1975) theorized that shame and insecurity, as well as rage and aggression, were underlying narcissism. Kernberg (1975) stressed the importance of timely interpretive work and the management of countertransferential issues. Kohut (1966) posited that the grandiose fantasies displayed by narcissistic individuals are repressed and not easily accessible. While these states are not easily modified by interactions in the patient's social world, the therapeutic relationship can uncover these processes and nurture a maturational process. Although debate continues about whether diverse theories reflect different patient presentations (Grenyer, 2013), there is increasing consensus about the different facets of personality pathology. It may be that the proponents of different therapeutic approaches emphasize different features (Gunderson et al., 2018). Early personality disorder theories are based on a medical model of disease (Livesley, 2018). These theories are characterized by an identifiable etiology, a number of pathogno-monic features, a threshold for differentiating normal from pathology, and a clear prognosis (Clark et al., 2017). These conceptualizations fall short of what we now know about personality disorders. The etiology of personality disorders is marked by complexity; vulnerability factors interact with precipitating factors, contributing to problems in domains of functioning (i.e., emotions, behaviors, interpersonal, sense of self; e.g., for BPD; Zanarini, 2019).

Personality disorders are heterogeneous disorders, meaning people have diverse presentations. Consequently, relying solely on a categorical perspective is problematic because it oversimplifies relevant information. When treating people with personality disorders, a diagnosis can be a useful starting point for guiding an overall treatment plan. However, contemporary efforts to guide treatment extend beyond general diagnoses and aim to increase specificity and levels of understanding. To address the limitations of a medical approach to conceptualizing personality disorder, Livesley (2018) recommended a conception of personality pathology that is anchored in an adaptive-evolutionary perspective, linked to normal personality development, and encourages the adoption of an integrative lens to understand different levels of conceptualization.

The medical approach to categorizing personality disorders has had a major impact on the field of personality disorders. Until the 1980s, mental health professionals, therapists, and theorists viewed personality disorders as problematic and "chronic." Psychological treatments were considered unhelpful (Lewis & Appleby, 1988). With the introduction of personality disorders in *DSM-III* (American Psychiatric Association, 1980), a number of specific categories were defined, including BPD (Widiger, 2018). This dramatic change to nosology fueled research and interest in the treatment of personality disorders. As the classification of personality disorders evolved and diagnoses became more reliable, it became increasingly easier to develop and study the efficacy of treatments.

The field of psychology has oscillated between conceptualizing personality in terms of traits (what personality "is") and functioning (what personality "does"; Allport, 1937). A descriptive approach to a phenomenon (e.g., "traits"; what it is) differs from an evaluative approach ("functioning"; what it serves). Research supports both conceptualizations. Functional aspects of personality depend on specific traits and their conglomeration (Nuzum et al., 2019), and they can be tied to the severity of a personality disorder, specifically BPD (Clark et al., 2018). When a person interacts with the environment, a complementarity exists between stable traits and their dynamic adaptive potential for functioning. Both approaches to conceptualization are part of the fifth edition text revision of the *Diagnostic and Statistical Manual of Mental Disorders* (5th ed., text rev.; *DSM-5-TR*) alternative model for personality disorder (American Psychiatric Association, 2022; see also the World Health Organization [WHO], 2022, for the *ICD-11*). According to WHO (2022), a personality disorder is characterized by "impairments in functioning of aspects of the self (e.g., identity, self-worth, capacity for self-direction) and/or problems in interpersonal functioning (e.g., developing and maintaining close and mutually satisfying relationships, understanding others' perspectives, managing conflict in relationships)" (Personality Disorders and Related Traits section, para.1). From this definition, it follows that treatment should focus on an individual's deviations from cultural expectations and on how an individual's functional patterns have become pervasive and inflexible across time.

With this background to conceptualizations of personality, psychotherapy researchers interested in personality disorders initially focused on countering the pessimistic view of personality disorders as chronic mental conditions. Historically, research by Linehan et al. (1991) on dialectical behavioral therapy (DBT) directly challenged pessimistic views of the treatability of BPD and helped fuel research on the effectiveness of treatment for personality disorders, particularly BPD. Today, dozens of well-conducted randomized controlled trials have established the efficacy of several specialized psychotherapeutic treatments designed specifically for BPD (Cristea et al., 2017; Storebø et al., 2020). They include DBT, transference-focused psychotherapy (Yeomans et al., 2015) and mentalization-based therapy (Bateman & Fonagy, 2015), schema therapy (Young, 2003), and others (e.g., cognitive analytic therapy, Systems Training for Emotional Predictability and Problem Solving, good psychiatric management). In line with the increased awareness of the treatability of BPD, researchers and clinicians working in developmental psychology and psychiatry have established that personality disorders also exist in adolescence (Chanen et al., 2017). This book will not focus on the treatment adaptations for adolescents, but interested readers may consult the growing literature on this topic. While the overall view of the treatability of BPD is positive, more work is needed to offer evidence on what treatment works for patients in a given context.

In the field of personality disorders, BPD has received far more attention than other personality disorders in the clinical and research literature. Decades of treatment research, mostly based on randomized controlled trial methodology, provide evidence that guides the treatment of BPD (Choi-Kain et al., 2017; Simonsen et al., 2019). Emerging evidence supports the efficacy of several treatment options for other personality disorders (Budge et al., 2013), such as narcissistic personality disorder (e.g., Ronningstam, 2020).

There have been longstanding beliefs about personality disorders, their psychopathology, and course. In the following section, we address two long-standing ideas about personality disorders and review relevant research that disputes these claims.

Claim 1: Personality Disorders Are Psychological and Not Somatic
Empirical evidence has shown that personality and personality disorders have neurobiological correlates and a diversity of etiopathogenetic pathways (Friedel & Stahl, 2018; Herpertz, 2013; MacNamara & Phan, 2018) and that functional domains associated with personality disorders have neurobiological underpinnings.

There is evidence of different functional domains associated with personality disorders. For example, aggression in males with BPD is underpinned by an activated left amygdala, as well as activation in the lateral orbitofrontal and dorsolateral prefrontal cortices in response to social rejection (Herpertz et al., 2017). Impulsive aggression is associated with dysfunction in three different neural networks: ventral prefrontal-amygdalar circuits (underlying fear learning), frontostriatal circuits (underlying reinforcement and cognitive learning), and frontoparietal circuits (involved in social cognition; Lee et al., 2018).

Emotional dysregulation involves deficits in the ability to distance from an emotional stimulus and engage in reappraisal strategies and may be associated with several neurofunctional activations in patients with BPD (Bertsch et al., 2018). For example, when instructed to distance themselves from an emotional stimulus, BPD patients, in comparison to healthy controls, showed higher levels of arousal in the insula and lower levels of activation in the left orbitofrontal cortex, the middle frontal gyrus, the left precuneus, the left middle temporal gyrus, the right superior temporal gyrus, and the right pallidum (Schulze et al., 2011).

Deficits in social cognition and the capacity to mentalize have been shown to be associated with neurofunctional networks, particularly the anterior medial prefrontal cortex, the temporoparietal junction, and several fronto-parietal networks (Herpertz, 2013; Lis et al., 2018; Luyten & Fonagy, 2018). When instructed to judge humorous stimuli involving the theory of mind, patients with BPD presented with a decreased functional connectivity between the anterior cingulate cortex and the left superior temporal regions, the right supramarginal and inferior parietal lobes, and the middle cingulate cortex (O'Neill et al., 2015). Insecure attachment has been shown to be associated with the development of the reward system in the brain (Luyten & Fonagy, 2018). Oxytocin has been found to have beneficial effects on affiliative behaviors in stressful situations (Neumann, 2009). While this research demonstrates that neuropeptides may contribute to functional prosocial behavior, these effects are specific to certain contexts. In help-seeking situations, increased affiliative behaviors are associated with oxytocin if the helper is from the out-group. Oxytocin has a mitigating effect on the help-seeker's prosocial behaviors and tends to increase interpersonal distrust and decrease cooperation (Bartz et al., 2011).

Claim 2: Personality Disorders Are Stable and Chronic

Contrary to early viewpoints, personality disorders, particularly BPD, are not stable over time. Longitudinal studies of the course of BPD reveal that person-ality pathology is not stable and that fluctuations in symptom clusters are the norm (Zanarini et al., 2016). However, stability in psychosocial functioning over time with fluctuations in identity and interpersonal behavior has been observed (Zanarini, 2019).

Several lines of research challenge the notion that personality itself is sta-ble. Current perspectives on personality research acknowledge some degree of sameness across situations but regard personality as a set of time-dependent phenomena that vary over time. This idea was initially put forth in Mischel's (1973) whole-trait theory and his description of structural aspects of person-ality. An implication of this viewpoint is that personality "trait" and "state" may describe, at least partially, the same behaviors (Fleeson et al., 2019). These perspectives on personality differ in that states are manifest and may be assessed over much shorter times than traits. Using the five-factor model of personality, Fleeson (2004) showed that the factor structure at the trait level was also found at the state level. This was determined using ecological momentary assessment to measure extraversion and rate how talkative the participant was in the past 15 minutes several times a day. What this research showed is that the same organization of traits was observed on the level of these supposedly fluctuating behaviors ("states") as on the level of the sup-posedly stable markers of the personality ("traits"). For clinical populations and particularly relevant for our purpose in this book, the same methods have been applied to examine the precipitants to symptoms in BPD. Fleeson and colleagues (2019) found that BPD symptoms fluctuate within short periods. For example, these studies found that dissociative symptoms were precipi-tated by negative affect, intense anger was precipitated by social rejection, interpersonal problems were precipitated by impulsivity, and antagonistic behavior was precipitated by perceived antagonistic behavior. These studies speak to a functional conception of states and traits in personality research.

Broader research on personality dynamics and structure also challenges the notion that personality is stable. Zimmermann et al. (2019) found consistency between a within-person approach to the assessing personality (i.e., day-by-day assessment) and a between-person approach. Interestingly, the five-factor trait domain model of the Personality Inventory for *DSM-5* (Krueger et al., 2012) fit diary-based data from both student samples and samples of hospitalized patients with psychological disorders.

Although we have highlighted that personality and personality disorders are fluid phenomena, several authors have found the use of syndromal or categorical descriptions still valuable for diagnostic purposes (e.g., Huprich, 2020). We argue that, when describing personality pathology, there are four functionally related levels of abstraction that are hierarchically nested (states, traits, syndromes, and categories of personality disorders; see Figure 2.1). In line with Fleeson's (2004) argument, categories of personality disorders represent the highest level of abstraction, which is consistent with all the other lower level abstractions. From a hierarchical nesting approach, states are on the lowest level of abstraction, after which are traits, then syndromal categories (Huprich, 2020; Ronningstam, 2020). Whether this hierarchy of abstraction shows full consistency across domains of personality needs to be evaluated in future research. At least for BPD, there seems to be a functional correspondence between categorical descriptors on the one hand and the description of psychopathology as trait and functioning (i.e., severity) on the other (Nuzum et al., 2019), but more research is needed in this area.

Let's illustrate these ideas with an example. Considering the functional domain of emotional dysregulation, emotion arousal varies from moment to moment within individuals and is highly influenced by the interpersonal context. Neurobiological activation in the functional network that links the amygdala, insula, and ventral striatum with the orbitofrontal cortex and the anterior cingulate cortex underpins emotional arousal when processing emotional tasks (MacNamara & Phan, 2018). This high within-subject fluctuation

FIGURE 2.1. Four Levels of Understanding of Problems Related to Personality Pathology

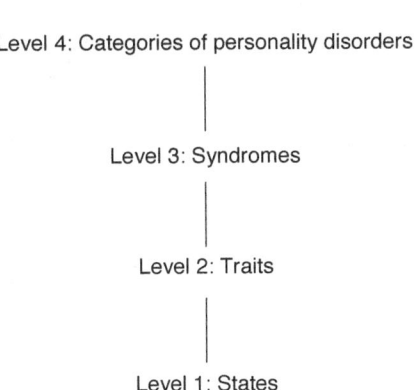

Level 4: Categories of personality disorders

Level 3: Syndromes

Level 2: Traits

Level 1: States

may be described on the level of between-subject variance as a problematic trait, such as the general propensity for increased negative affectivity. Such negative affectivity traits may emerge in a stable pattern in response to interpersonal situations, such as hypersensitivity to social rejection, which may be found on the level of a between-subject apparently stable syndrome. Finally, together with other observed syndromes, the latter compose a distinct personality disorder, such as BPD or narcissistic personality disorder, on the level of a categorical conception. The process-based fluid conception of personality pathology may be the moment-by-moment "microlevel" correspondent of the traditional "macrolevel" distinctions where individuals are differentiated among themselves as a function of categories, syndromes, and traits.

In conclusion, we offer the perspective that the conceptualization of personality disorders in adults will evolve into one of a fluid, process-based organization of functional domains associated with personality pathology.

A FUNCTIONAL DOMAIN PERSPECTIVE

Personality disorders can be viewed in terms of a number of functional domains. A *functional domain* refers to specific problematic patterns of responses that are manifest at the state, trait, and syndromal levels of psychopathology and are embedded in an evolutionary-adaptive framework. A functional domain represents pathognomonic features of personality disorders. Functional domains cut across all levels of conceptualization of personality and bridge neurobiological and psychological substrates. They translate the severity—functional—perspective of personality disorders into clinically relevant descriptive trait domains. They may be regarded as an important focus of treatment interventions. Functional domains allow for a description of the mechanism of etiology and mechanism of dysfunction. Domains of functioning can explain psychopathology and resilience. The functional domain can be studied at any of these levels using psychological and/or neurobiological methods.

Functional domains are similar, though they can be distinguished from the definition of dimensions put forward by the National Institute of Mental Health's Research Domain Criteria (RDoC; Clark et al., 2017; Hyman, 2010), which was conceived to stimulate research in mental health and encourage multidisciplinary research and the integration of a biological and psychological approach to the study of a clinical problem. Functional domains may help advance the study of psychopathology and mental health by taking into account multilevel complexity. The RDoC dimensions include negative valence (responsible for responses to aversion, such as threat or loss), positive valence (responsible for responses related to reward), cognitive system (responsible for control, attention, and memory), social processes (responsible for communication, attachment, and affiliation), and arousal (responsible for modulatory responses and circadian rhythms). The developers of RDoC hoped that this system would offer a structured framework for novel research perspectives and be supportive of the development of new methodologies (in psychometrics, physiology, and neurobiology), ultimately leading to the development of more precise assessment methods in psychopathology and even more personalized treatment.

A functional domain, as we understand it, also differs from the trait domains conceptualized in the alternative model of personality disorders described in *DSM-5-TR* and the domains described in *ICD-11* (Clark et al., 2018). Functional and trait domains aim to synthesize a range of responses into a coherent pattern. Our functional domain perspective is akin to what personality "does," or its impact on functioning, rather than taking a descriptive approach. Finally, a functional domain also differs from traits because they are classified by an emerging Hierarchical Taxonomy of Psychopathology (HiTOP) framework (Ruggero et al., 2019). A hierarchical classification offers a transdiagnostic perspective of the structure of psychopathology, whereas functional domains do not cover the full array of psychopathology. Functional domains are major hubs for change. They imply that there are fruitful opportunities for change incorporated within them, which can be used as starting points to personalize treatment. Functional domains describe potential impactful features of personality on human interactions—and aim at describing the functional effects on interactions—while traits are solely descriptors organized without necessarily a functional perspective (but rather based on co-occurrence between traits).

In this book, we focus on five central functional domains: emotional dysregulation, disturbed social interaction, identity problems, impulsivity, and cognitive disturbances.

Emotional Dysregulation

Emotional dysregulation is a core problem characterizing BPD (Linehan et al., 2007), other personality disorders (e.g., Ronningstam, 2016), and other mental health problems (McMain et al., 2010). Ochsner and Gross (2005) proposed a model of emotion regulation described as a multistep salutogenic process involving cognitive appraisal and reappraisal, followed by coping responses. At each step in the process, emotion modulation can occur. Emotion regulation plays a functional role on various levels day by day.

Several studies have shown that individuals with BPD compared with healthy controls have deficits in cognitive appraisal (Sauer-Zavala et al.,

2016) and use dysfunctional coping strategies (Kramer, 2014). Moreover, individuals with BPD exhibit an increased responsivity to stress-related stimuli, high avoidance of emotional experience in the present, and suppressed positively and negatively valenced emotions (Beblo et al., 2013). Emotional dysregulation has a negative impact on interpersonal relationships, including the therapeutic relationship.

Emotional lability in BPD is a core feature of the disorder, and several studies have used ecological momentary assessment to examine emotional lability. After reviewing the empirical data on the stability of emotional states in samples, including many individuals diagnosed with BPD, Santangelo et al. (2014) found that these individuals experienced extreme and rapid shifts in emotions and fluctuated between positive and negative emotions every day. Fluctuations in emotions were much stronger for individuals with BPD than healthy controls. In another study, Harpøth et al. (2021) found that patients' daily self-reported positive emotions predicted quality of life and ego resilience prospectively on the following day. In addition, positive emotions had a greater impact on resilience than negative emotions.

Emotional dysregulation has been found to be linked to specific neurofunctional pathways in the brain. Dysfunctional appraisal processes are associated with decreased orbitofrontal and increased insular activity (Bertsch et al., 2018). In addition, hyperarousal is associated with increased activation in the amygdala (Schulze et al., 2016). There is evidence that, compared with healthy controls, individuals with BPD show no differences in reactivity. Emotional dysregulation was accounted for by abnormal baseline functioning, as indicated by elevated heart rate and reduced sinus arrhythmia (Kuo et al., 2016). In another study, individuals with BPD showed higher sympathetic arousal and lower vagal tonus than healthy controls (Kuo & Linehan, 2009). Deficits in modulatory pathways linked to the prefrontal cortex and amygdala have been associated with emotional dysregulation in personality disorders (e.g., New et al., 2007; Silbersweig et al., 2007; Silvers et al., 2017). Deficits in emotion modulation are more likely to be exhibited in response to negative interpersonal stimuli (e.g., social exclusion, facial emotion expression) rather than general negative stimuli.

Disturbed Social Interaction

Disturbed social interaction is a characteristic of several categories of personality disorders, particularly BPD. Difficult social interaction may go beyond specific interpersonally "manipulative" strategies (Bland & Rossen, 2005) but may involve a host of underlying social-cognitive processes at play when the individual interacts with a social partner, including close relationships, attachment figures, occasional strangers, and of course, the psychotherapist. Disturbed social interactions include activated difficulties in perspective taking and developing emotional and cognitive empathy for the other's experience and specific disturbances in theory of mind, mentalizing, and metacognitive abilities. Interestingly, studies have demonstrated a lack of disturbed social cognition in personality disorders (e.g., BPD, antisocial personality disorder, schizotypal personality disorder; Lis et al., 2018; Schnell & Herpertz, 2018), and empirical arguments have shown that certain patients with BPD may actually outperform healthy controls on specific laboratory tasks related to social cognition (Fertuck et al., 2009). This differentiated picture calls for a rigorous definition but may also represent some of the clinical variation found in patients with BPD; through difficult or traumatic interactions in the past, some of these patients may have learned to cope by developing outstanding capacities of mind reading and perspective taking.

A particularly interesting feature underlying social interaction is the difficulty observed in many patients with BPD (and other personality disorders) to form a trusting relationship. Trust may take different forms: trust in knowledge transmitted by the other (Fonagy et al., 2015), trust in oneself as a reliable resource of information, trust in the other as a caring person, and trust in one's capacity to be effective (Signer et al., 2020). These aspects of trust can potentially influence the psychotherapeutic process and outcome. Clinically, patients with BPD present with typical interpersonal patterns, as defined by the core conflictual relationship theme case formulation method. Drapeau et al. (2012) found that patients with BPD may present with interactions that highlight an ego-ideal, a dependent-depressive interaction (e.g., "I wish to be dependent, the other is self-conscious, and I feel depressed"), a passive-submissive interaction pattern, or sadomasochistic interaction (e.g., "I wish to be hurt, the other is not accepting, and I feel guilty"). It remains an open question whether these capacities and observations are stable and resourceful functions over time.

Sadikaj et al. (2013) compared the emergence of quarrelsome behaviors in daily life between patients with BPD and healthy controls. The researchers asked questions pertaining to three different sociocognitive processes that take place within the person: behavioral reactivity to interpersonal perceptions, affect reactivity to interpersonal perceptions, and behavioral reactivity to a person's own affect. Interestingly, while the latter did not differ between patients with BPD and healthy controls, the former two predicted the emergence of quarrelsomeness. That is, when patients with BPD perceive others as cold or vindicative, their interpersonal behavior a few hours later is then reliably more quarrelsome, and they feel an increased level of negative affect.

Difficult social interaction involves a variety of neurofunctional domains and areas in the brain, the study of which related to personality disorders has just begun. One of the subfunctions that has received attention is the theory of mind, a domain associated with activation in the anterior medial prefrontal cortex and the temporoparietal junction. Patients with schizotypal personality disorder present with difficulty putting themselves into the mind of another and fail to recognize emotions in others; these difficulties are similar to those observed in schizophrenia (see Dickey et al., 2002) and autism (Perez-Rodriguez et al., 2014) in terms of the neurobiological underpinnings.

For patients with BPD, structures such as the superior temporal gyrus and the superior temporal sulcus were associated with difficulty performing tasks involving recruiting a theory of mind (Dziobek et al., 2011). A reduced functional coupling was observed between these theory-of-mind neural networks and those responsible for emotion regulation (O'Neill et al., 2015). Overinterpreting social cues—a function associated with errors in mentalizing—was associated with BPD when these patients were invited to play a trust game involving virtual interaction partners who seemed either more or less untrustworthy (King-Casas et al., 2008). The researchers found difficulty in developing collaboration, which they explained by a lack of understanding of social cues; this may be linked with the observed lack of modulation in the insula in response to the interaction partners' bids in the game. Despite the complexity of the construct, we can report that disturbed social interactions have cognitive, affective, and neurofunctional underpinnings.

Identity Problems

Identity diffusion and problems related to identity are core features of personality disorders, particularly the most severe ones, especially BPD (Jorgensen, 2018). Livesley (2003) defined identity problems as the "failure to establish stable and integrated representations of self and others" (p. 19). While problems in identity development may be mostly associated with adolescence and young adulthood, identity formation is an ongoing developmental task during the entire lifespan (see also Lind et al., 2019, 2022). Without discussing in detail the rich literature on identity and problematic identity processes, it is noteworthy that the latter are now part of the alternative model for *DSM-5-TR* (p. 762; American Psychiatric Association, 2022) as part of personality functioning, defined as functioning with stable limits within a person and with others and marked with a stable sense of self over time. Identity diffusion and the healthy development of the self emerge as a complex, multifaceted process marked by (dis)integration. As Kernberg (1984) noted, it is important to consider identity as a complex construction process involving the individual's affective, or emotional, experience.

Beeney et al. (2015) found that individuals diagnosed with BPD had high levels of unstable and negative self-representations. Using a card-sorting task, these researchers found that individuals with BPD sorted self-aspects using a higher proportion of negative traits, evidenced less integrated sorts, and showed less consistency in self-concept over a 3-hour period. These findings were associated with activation in brain regions using functional magnetic resonance imaging. Individuals with BPD had high levels of activation in the precuneus and posterior cingulate when reflecting on the self. Steiner et al. (2021) found that individuals characterized by high levels of narcissism developed a composite of themselves that was rated as significantly more attractive than their actual image. Research on college students supports the importance of identity processes in the link between negative affectivity and the urge to self-harm (Lear & Pepper, 2016). It remains an open question as to how these aspects play out from a functional domain perspective.

In a study using ecological momentary assessment, Scala et al. (2018) showed that items pertaining to the self, negative affectivity, and identity explained the day-to-day urges for self-harming behaviors in BPD. Specifically, high self-concept clarity—the internal consistency and stability over time of clearly defined beliefs about the self—played the role of a resource, or buffer, in the link between negative affectivity and urges to self-harm. Only when the self-concept clarity was low—which was interpreted as identity disturbance—was negative affectivity linked with self-harm urges. Interestingly, this model was robust for both BPD and anxiety disorder.

Impulsivity

Impulsive acts are part of the diagnostic criteria of BPD, and impulsivity is part of the alternative model of the *DSM-5-TR* personality disorder trait domain of disinhibition. *Impulsivity* may be defined as a rash action under stress without taking into account its negative consequences. Impulsivity is generally oriented toward the self (i.e., self-harm, suicidal thoughts and acts) and others (the latter being impulsive aggression), in addition to other impulsive patterns (Zanarini, 2019). While these symptoms may be understood as one of the prototypical expressions of the acute symptoms of BPD, the underlying determinants of impulsive urges, thoughts, and behaviors are much broader. The use of impulsive behaviors to respond to interpersonally stressful situations, regulate emotions (particularly unacknowledged fear), interrupt cognitive disturbance or dissociation, and find some "comfort" in the subjectively well-known self-harming behavior (explaining the addictive potential of the latter) have been described in the literature (e.g., Kleindienst et al., 2008).

Impulsivity is a multidimensional construct that has long been associated with personality disorders, particularly with BPD and antisocial personality disorder. Broadly, impulsivity is conceptualized in terms of deficits in inhibitory control, resulting in an inability to suppress responses leading to undesirable consequences. Early research on impulsivity was largely based on self-report measures of impulsivity. For example, the Barratt Impulsiveness Scale (BIS-11; Patton et al., 1995) is one of the most widely used self-report measures of impulsivity that assesses its three dimensions: attentional impulsiveness, motor impulsiveness, and nonplanning impulsiveness. Behavioral, neurobiological, and cognitive research has led to advancements in understanding the multidimensional nature of impulsivity. There is a current movement to abandon general measures of impulsivity and adopt a more precise definition of impulsivity, along with its specific phenotypes (Bari et al., 2016).

Berenson et al. (2011) discussed a specific dynamic contingency in relation to impulsivity in the daily life of BPD. The study used ecological momentary assessment to explain the emergence of rage in the daily life of persons with BPD. The researchers found a high average and fluctuation of problematic perception of social rejection in individuals with BPD, unlike in healthy controls. The intensity of perceived social rejection by the individual explained rage in BPD but not in healthy controls (Berenson et al., 2011).

Impulsivity recruits three neurobiological circuits associated with personality disorders (Lee et al., 2018). The first circuit regulates fear learning and passes through the amygdala and the ventral prefrontal areas. The second circuit hosts the principle related to reinforcement and involves the striatum and the orbitofrontal and cingulate cortex. The third circuit builds directly on social cognition and involves the frontoparietal networks, particularly the precuneus, medial prefrontal cortex, and temporoparietal junction.

Impulsivity, particularly impulsive aggression, may be understood as a functional domain built on some of the features related to disturbed social interaction (as described earlier). This is relevant for the social information processing model, in which the impulsive act depends on a series of sequences, particularly the encoding of social information (i.e., perception and interpretation of facial expressions in the other indexes of social rejection).

Impulse control problems in people diagnosed with personality disorders may arise from several neurobiological mechanisms. There is consistent evidence showing that motor impulsivity involves neurocircuits in the interior frontal cortex (McHugh & Balaratnasingam, 2018; Sebastian et al., 2014). Deficits in inhibitory control have been shown to worsen under stress (McHugh & Balaratnasingam, 2018; Sebastian et al., 2014). Motor impulsivity has also been associated with decreased activity in the orbitofrontal cortex, which is involved in executive functioning regulating decision making (Kaplan et al., 2020). Furthermore, aggressive impulsivity in personality disorders is associated with reduced prefrontal cortex inhibition and the suppression of limbic activity in response to emotional provocation or threat cues (Siever & Weinstein, 2009).

Studies have shown that in personality disorders, the prefrontal cortex, which has been linked to social judgments and emotional evaluation, is not efficiently used to suppress limbic activity that generates aggression (Siever & Weinstein, 2009). Finally, research has shown that impulsive behavior in personality disorders may arise from abnormalities in the frontal-limbic networks, including the anterior cingulate cortex.

Cognitive Disturbances

The final functional domain concerns cognitive disturbances, which include usual beliefs and experiences, eccentricity, and cognitive and perceptual dysregulation (including dissociation). They are summarized in the *DSM-5-TR* under the trait domain of psychoticism versus lucidity (American Psychiatric Association, 2022). The stress-related transient emergence of paranoid ideation or severe dissociative states is one of nine diagnostic criteria for BPD. While the nature of the phenomenon may be shared with schizophrenia, the content and transience of the cognitive dysregulatory states are specific to personality disorders, particularly BPD (Zanarini, 2009). From a functional perspective, the description and study of these phenomena and when they occur in real life remain highly challenging.

Glaser et al. (2010) systematically described transient cognitive dysregulation in BPD using ecological momentary assessment. The researchers compared cognitive dysregulation in response to stress in daily life between individuals with BPD, individuals with other Cluster C personality disorders (i.e., dependent, avoidant, obsessive-compulsive personality disorders), individuals with psychotic disorders, and controls. While the increase in paranoid ideation was comparable across all groups facing stress, individuals with BPD had the strongest overall reactivity in terms of the increase in cognitive dysregulation in response to stress in daily life. It is interesting to note that cognitive dysregulation pertaining to BPD may not only involve dissociation and paranoia but also, as shown in this study, a variety of state-dependent hallucinations generally related to psychotic experiences.

These five functional domains may be assessed using self-report questionnaires, observer-rated scales, or clinician-rated assessments and interviews, which may be relevant for both research and practice. A nonexhaustive list of measures, scales, and subscales, per functional domain and assessment perspective, are compiled in Table 2.1. Because this conception is fundamentally anchored in the dimensional conception of personality disorders, we globally recommend the assessment tools developed or currently in development, for personality pathology according to the *DSM-5-TR* and the *ICD-11* (for a

TABLE 2.1. Possible Assessment Tools of the Five Functional Domains in Personality Pathology

Functional domains	Self-report tools	Observer-rated tools	Clinician-rated interviews
Emotional dysregulation	SCID-AMPD subscale Negative Affectivity DABS DBT-WCCL DERS DTS KIMS PID-5-BF PROMIS subscale Positive SAM	CAP-RS CEAS-R O-MAR	DABS subscale Negative affectivity SCID-AMPD
Social interaction problems	IIP IMI-R NTB PROMIS subscale Social RFQ A-RSQ SCS-R SNI UCLA	BIBS subscale Interpersonal CCRT MAS-R RF-RS SI-BPD	DIB-R subscale Interpersonal

Construct			
Identity problems	No tools available	AIQ DSS MLQ RSES SCCS	SCID-AMPD subscale Identity STIPO
Impulsivity	No tools available	BIS PID-5-BF subscale Impulsivity UPPS-P	DIB-R subscale Impulsivity SCID-AMPD subscale Impulsivity
Cognitive disturbances	NEPCS	PID-5 subscale Psychoticism	DIB-R subscale Cognition SCID-AMPD subscale Psychoticism

Note. AIQ = Aspects of Identity Questionnaire (Cheek & Briggs, 2013); A-RSQ = Adult Rejection Sensitivity Questionnaire (Berenson et al., 2013); BIBS = Beziehungs-Interaktions- Bearbeitungsskalen (Sachse et al., 2015); BIS = Barratt Impulsiveness Scale (Patton et al., 1995); CAP-RS = Coping Action Patterns–Rating System (Perry et al., 2005); CCRT = Core Conflictual Relationship Theme (Luborsky & Crits-Christoph, 1998); CEAS-R = Client Emotional Arousal Scale-Revised (Warwar & Greenberg, 1999); DABS = Derogatis Affects Balance Scale (Derogatis, 1975); DBT-WCCL = Dialectical Behavior Therapy Ways of Coping Checklist (Neacsiu, Rizvi, & Linehan, 2010); DERS = Dimensions of Emotion Regulation Scale (Gratz & Roemer, 2004); DIB-R = Diagnostic Interview for Borderlines-Revised (Zanarini et al., 1989); DSS = Dissociative Symptoms Scale (Carlson et al., 2018); DTS = Distress Tolerance Scale (Simons & Gaher, 2005); IIP = Inventory of Interpersonal Problems (Horowitz et al., 1988); IMI-R = Impact Message Inventory-Revised (Kiesler & Schmidt, 2006); KIMS = Kentucky Inventory of Mindfulness Scale (Baer et al., 2004); MAS-R = Meta-Cognitive Assessment Scale-Revised (Carcione et al., 2010); MLQ = Meaning of Life Questionnaire (Steger et al., 2006); NTB = Need to Belong Scale (Leary, 2013); NEPCS = Narrative-Emotion Process Coding System 2.0 (Angus et al., 2017); O-MAR = Observer-Rated Measure of Affect Regulation (Watson & Prosser, 2004); PID-5-BF = Personality Inventory for *DSM-5*-Brief Form (Krueger et al., 2013); PROMIS = Patient-Reported Outcomes Measurement Information System (U.S. Department of Health and Human Services, 2023); RF-RS = Reflexive-Function (Fonagy et al., 1998); RFQ = Reflective Functioning Questionnaire (Fonagy et al., 2016); RSES = Rosenberg Self-Esteem Scale (Rosenberg, 1965); SAM = Self-Assessment Manikin (Bradley & Lang, 1994); SCCS = Self-Concept Clarity Scale (Campbell et al., 1996); SCID-AMPD = Structured Clinical Interview for the *DSM-5* Alternative Model of Personality Disorder (Skodol et al., 2018); SCS-R = Social Connectedness Scale-Revised (Lee et al., 2001); SI-BPD = Social interaction problems in BPD (Signer et al., 2020); SNI = Social Network Index (subscales Interpersonal Distance and Trust; Berkman & Syme, 1979); STIPO = Structured Interview of Personality Organization (Clarkin, Caligor, et al., 2007); UCLA = UCLA Loneliness Scale (Russell et al., 1978); UPPS-P = Urgency, Premeditation, Perseverance, Sensation Seeking, and Positive Urgency Impulsive Behavior Scale (Whiteside & Lynam, 2001). Impulsivity and lack of inhibitory control is typically assessed using neuropsychological tests (go-no-go, Connors Continuous Performance Test-3 [Kao & Thomas, 2010] not in the table).

review, see Bach et al., 2020). Of note, in the context of this book and to save space, we offer this nonexhaustive list without discussing the exact levels of validity, fidelity, and reliability of each measure. We invite you to consult the scientific literature cited to gain knowledge about the psychometric properties of each assessment tool before applying it in research and practice.

In this book, we address these five functional domains and discuss additional clinical problems that are central to therapeutic work with patients with personality disorders. A word of caution is needed here. While the book focuses on personality disorders in general, we admit that most research has focused on BPD. This inequivalence of evidence is inevitably reflected in the research elaborations in this book. Another caveat is needed in regard to the presented empirical studies in the field of BPD (and of personality disorders more general). We discussed the great heterogeneity of BPD, but in the nomothetic research designs, this heterogeneity is rarely accounted for. Finally, we must acknowledge that the formal comparison between BPD and healthy controls does not provide information about the specificity of BPD but rather speaks to the general deficits related to psychopathology; more specific comparisons with other clinical groups are needed.

In what follows, in addition to discussing mechanisms of change anchored in the five functional domains, we discuss difficulties in the therapeutic relationship (see Chapter 9) and during the first contact (see Chapter 3), which represent key clinical tasks in psychotherapies for personality disorders.

CONCLUSIONS

Therapeutic work with patients with personality pathology requires a multifaceted and consistent theoretical context informed by empirical evidence and clinical wisdom. In light of the debate between the proponents of the categorical model of personality disorders and proponents of dimensional conceptions, the actual functional underpinnings of the pathological process are often overlooked. We argue that it is fruitful to conceptualize personality pathology within a limited number of functional domains informed by empirical evidence on psychological and neurobiological levels and clinical wisdom. We suggest these are emotional dysregulation, disturbed social interaction, identity problems, impulsivity, and cognitive disturbances. Activated behaviors associated with a functional domain become opportunities for profound and lasting change through psychotherapy. As such, these may become target domains— which may, if treated, yield intermediate outcomes—in psychotherapy that is informed by mechanisms of change.

3

THE FIRST SESSION OF PSYCHOTHERAPY AND GETTING STARTED IN TREATMENT

This chapter addresses the topic of how to begin treatment with a patient presenting with a personality disorder. We discuss how to get things off to a strong start in the first session. We address how to develop a treatment focus and a clear frame and how to address and prevent therapy-interfering behaviors. All this is predicated on a sound case formulation to understand and guide the therapy process. We know that case formulation may have an impact on the therapy process and outcome. It may further the therapist's clarity about potential explanations of a manifest behavior and assist them with treatment planning. Other essential therapist activities in the first session include assessment, developing a positive relationship by listening, responding empathically, conveying validation, expressing warmth, and developing a focus for the treatment. The first session needs to engage the patient, increasing their motivation to change while mitigating the risks of dropout. All these tasks are relevant to the therapeutic work for patients with a personality disorder and represent the groundwork for a focus on mechanisms of change in psychotherapy.

This chapter is the first that delves into clinical challenges from an event-based perspective. We describe common clinical problems occurring during

https://doi.org/10.1037/0000388-004
Understanding Mechanisms of Change in Psychotherapies for Personality Disorders, by U. Kramer, K. N. Levy, and S. McMain

the first contact with a patient with a personality disorder. Facing these clinical problems or challenging events, we propose solutions that we believe, from our theoretical perspectives, can be implemented by any therapist, independently of the treatment modality and theory. Note that several topics pertaining to the initial session are also discussed in-depth throughout the book, where more recommendations may be found.

TYPICAL CHALLENGES ENCOUNTERED IN THE FIRST SESSION AND HOW THERAPISTS CAN RESPOND

Getting started on the right foot in therapy is not easy for therapists when working with patients with personality disorders. To facilitate a good start, we present several typical clinical challenges and behaviors that can interfere with treatment from the outset. These challenges include (a) difficulties with therapeutic collaboration and trust, (b) criticism of the therapist, (c) display of suicidal and self-harming behavior and impulsivity, and (d) noncompliance with the treatment. These four challenging domains can be formulated as choice points or opportunities for change. We draw on clinical material to illustrate the challenges and discuss solutions.

Problems With Therapeutic Collaboration and Trust

What should the therapist do when the patient presents at the first session and refuses to sit down and communicate?

Such situations are not uncommon. Low levels of trust and nonengagement with the therapist is an ever-present problem, especially for patients with personality disorders. Low levels of trust and poor engagement with the therapist can take many forms. For example, a patient can arrive, refuse to sit down, and appear uncomfortable, choosing to stand throughout the session. In other situations, patients attend the session but quickly declare that they do not intend to stay, or they become upset and decide precipitously to leave. Or they threaten to leave, as in the case of a young man who entered the first meeting and, before the therapist could share any welcome, stated that if the therapist asked anything about his childhood, "I am out of here." When the therapist asked if he could say more about his concern, the patient angrily lectured about the irrelevance of childhood experiences with parents and maintained that only current relationships are important. Contrary to the patient's assumption, the therapist was interested in hearing about the current relationship difficulties before talking about developmental history. Thus, a therapist stance of acceptance, with a dose of genuine interest in the patient's experience, often helps in this situation.

What should the therapist do when the patient expresses concerns about the limits of confidentiality?

Concerns about the limits of confidentiality may arise in response to the therapist seeking to obtain collateral information from significant others, previous therapists, or physicians or in response to requests to audiotape or videotape for supervision purposes. In addition, this concern may be expressed by withholding certain information during the session. In regard to signing consent to speak with others, it is often best not to overly support and validate the patient's reluctance, although some validation may be appropriate. Rather than saying, "Of course, I understand," or "Of course, I would feel the same way," both of which may be true, it may be better to simply say something such as, "It is not uncommon that people have concerns—can you tell me about yours?" or even more simply, "Can you tell me about your concerns?" Both of these statements convey validation. It is normal to have concerns about confidentiality—most people do. Therapists should respect the patient's concern and seek to understand them better. In one situation, a patient was reluctant to let the therapist speak with a spouse. When the therapist asked about the patient's concern, the patient explained that their spouse was charming and convincing and they were afraid the therapist would be unduly influenced by the spouse's perspective and would no longer be on the patient's "side." The patient was afraid that the therapist would blame them for the marital problems and take their spouse's side. Similar dynamics can occur when speaking with adolescents and young adults in relation to parents and guardians. It is helpful to discuss explicitly what will be shared and what will not be shared with the patient's parents.

Of course, there are limitations to confidentiality in any therapy (e.g., suicidality, homicidality, threats of violence, child and/or elder abuse, risk of subpoena), and these limitations vary as a function of the legal situation in each country. Adolescents can have concerns about the therapist sharing information about drug use and/or sexual behavior. Spouses can have concerns about sharing information about infidelity or divorce intentions.

Patients may have concerns about what previous therapists may say. For example, one patient was adamant about not allowing a therapist or the clinic to communicate with his previous therapists, psychiatrists, and physicians despite the relevance of this information. Although the patient's concern was eventually expressed directly, they first communicated their concerns in an indirect and ambiguous manner and repeatedly failed to sign release forms. It is helpful to directly explore any concerns that are directly or indirectly raised. In this situation, the therapist explored the patient's concerns, leading the patient to acknowledge their fear that previous therapists would negatively influence the views of their current therapist. The patient felt that the previous therapist had doubts about the patient's concerns, and raising these concerns would create similar doubts for the current therapist. With a bit of exploration, it became apparent that the patient had doubts and wondered about their sensitivity, tendency to exaggerate, and even present physical complaints in ways that belied their authenticity. Once these concerns were directly verbalized, they could be addressed and the therapist's fear reduced, and the patient was eventually willing to sign the release.

What should a therapist do when a patient appears to leave things out or not disclose personal information?

At times, patients will conceal significant information and not disclose personal information. For example, the therapist might ask a direct question, to which the patient may respond that they do not know how to respond. Is this patient unable or unwilling to respond? In such situations, it may be necessary to clarify first whether the patient has understood the question and have them summarize what they understood. Then, it can be helpful to ask the patient if they do not know how to respond or if they would prefer not to share information—possibly even if they may have concerns about the therapist's reaction. Often, patients acknowledge they are concerned about what the therapist might think of them or that the therapist might judge them for their response. It can be useful for the therapist to normalize the patient's response. It is not uncommon for people to not want to disclose information that may illicit feelings of shame. Usually, a brief discussion of these worries can free up the patient and increase their willingness to be open.

When a patient sits back, does not share any information, and appears to wait for the therapist to begin the session, the therapist can respond in several ways. On the one hand, it is the patient's responsibility to begin the session, and doing so should be part of the frame to which the patient and therapist agree. On the other hand, it is the therapist's responsibility to engage and motivate the patient in treatment. When setting the treatment frame, the agreement should make each participant's roles and responsibilities clear so that when the patient deviates from the agreement, it can be discussed. If the patient does not begin the session, the therapist may ask, "So, what is on your mind?" This prompt is consistent with and reminds the patient of the initial agreement (if there is any in place yet). However, a patient sometimes responds by indicating there is nothing on their mind or with silence. If the patient indicates there is nothing on their mind, the therapist usually acknowledges that, at times, it can be difficult to start a session and instructs them to take a few minutes to reflect and see if something comes to mind. If the patient still indicates that nothing is coming to mind, the therapist might wonder to themselves if the absence of material is an indication that the patient is consciously suppressing important material. To test this idea, the therapist usually responds by asking the patient if there is nothing on their mind or if there is but there is some concern about sharing it with the therapist (or concern about what the therapist might think). The therapist should do this if the patient withholding important material is the central issue, taking precedence over other issues except suicidality, homicidality, or threats to the treatment.

What should the therapist do if the patient repeatedly seems to ignore their question or intervention in the first session?

If the therapist asks a question or asks for clarification and the patient is evasive, changes the topic, or responds as if the therapist asked a different question, it is useful to directly examine what is happening in that moment. The therapist can do this in a low-affect, matter-of-fact way rather than in an accusatory manner. The patient may be perplexed and unaware of what the therapist is referring to. The therapist might ask what is happening in the moment to slow the process down and give the patient time to reflect. We recommend using what may be called "parts language" to acknowledge the multiple aspects of the patient's experience. For example, the therapist might note how they recognize that the patient is putting in an effort to be attentive and responsive to their questions. However, the therapist might also note that, at the same time, it seems like there might be something difficult about the question just asked. The therapist can point out that maybe they are wrong and misperceiving things but then elaborate on how they are coming to that conclusion. For instance, the therapist might note they asked several times about a particular issue. The therapist should try not to make it about getting the answer to the question they asked but instead reflecting on the process. We find that when we understand what is getting in the way of the patient wanting to answer the question, it becomes easier to answer the question. It is important to recognize that, typically, one part of the patient wants to trust the therapist and collaborate, but another part is concerned about sharing the answer to the question asked.

What should the therapist do if the patient attempts to control the agenda (e.g., by talking excessively or remaining uncommunicative and refusing to respond or engage in dialogue)?

Like the previous question, the therapist may bring attention to the problem and help the patient reflect on what is happening. The therapist may begin by asking if the patient noticed their behavior. It is useful for the therapist to bring attention to the problem in the current interaction. The therapist can use their demeanor, tone, and phrasing to convey openness to being wrong, as the therapist wonders with the patient about what might be going on. A typical interpretation might start with acknowledging the patient's desire to engage in the therapy, illustrated by their being at therapy and sharing openly with the therapist. The therapist may then wonder if the patient might be anxious and making it difficult to allow the therapist to talk or ask questions. On the one hand, they may want help, but on the other hand, they are afraid of what the therapist might have to offer. Maybe they are afraid the therapist will impose their view on them, or maybe they are afraid that despite the therapist's best efforts, they will not be able to help them. Another possibility is that they are concerned the therapist is not truly interested in helping them. The therapist can use the content the patient has already shared and whatever else comes up in their discussion of what is happening to generate an initial hypothesis in the context of their case formulation, along with reasonable alternatives.

Responding to Criticism of the Therapist or of the Treatment

What should the therapist do when a patient criticizes the therapist for offering to meet for a few orientation sessions?

The patient may begin the first session by urgently stating, "I feel so much pain; I really want to get rid of this as quickly as possible." The therapist may acknowledge the pain and anxiety that appears to underlie the patient's remark. In addition to acknowledging the patient's distress and sense of urgency, the therapist may respond by orienting to the process of getting started in therapy. This can include discussing the patient's goals and history of problems and proposing a treatment plan so that the patient can make a well-informed decision. If a formal assessment has not already been conducted, the therapist may assess the scope and nature of the patient's difficulties and ask the patient to describe a specific distressing situation in their daily life. The first few orientation sessions can have therapeutic effects and can promote change.

What should the therapist do if the patient criticizes the therapist's appearance in the first session (e.g., their gender, age, or perceived race or ethnicity)?

A patient may say to a trainee therapist, "You look too young to have a PhD," "Am I your first patient?" or "Have you ever had a patient as difficult as me?" An inexperienced therapist may feel overwhelmed and anxious. It may be true that the therapist has never had a patient with borderline personality disorder (BPD). Generally, it is not recommended that trainees begin their training with challenging patients with personality disorders. In this situation, therapists need to modulate their reactions to the criticism. Then, irrespective of the trainee's stage of training, the therapist should try to understand what is driving the patient's comment, which may reflect something about the patient. The patient's comment may be motivated by a desire to appear excessively complex, possibly to ensure a rigorous course of treatment (e.g., questioning the trainee's credentials). It may also be driven by a fear of being overlooked or a desire to be seen as special to enlist extra support from the therapist. Based on hypotheses about the driving factors, the therapist could respond to the patient's unexpressed emotional need by saying, "Yes, I may look young, and I really appreciate you asking about my training. It sounds like it is really important for you to make sure that you get the best treatment, given the struggles you're experiencing. If you agree to engage in this therapy, I'll do my best to help you overcome your difficulties." The therapist may avoid acting in a complementary manner to the content of the patient's comments and instead respond in a complementary manner to the factors underlying the explicit comment.

Questions about age and credentials need to be addressed directly. However, when a patient asks about a therapist's age, it is not always evident that they are seeking a direct answer. Inquiries about the therapist's age can be driven by many factors. It could reflect an expression of concern about the therapist's competence. It can be helpful to ask a simple clarifying question such as, "Can you tell me more about your concern?" Therapists—especially inexperienced ones—may be reluctant to explore this concern. However, doing so conveys to the patient that it is safe to discuss such concerns. Sometimes, reference to the therapist's age may be linked to the patient's shame and envy of the therapist (e.g., envy of their youth, having their whole life ahead of them, being someone who has not wasted years). Older therapists may be viewed enviously as people who have successfully navigated developmental challenges or, conversely, may be perceived as being out of touch.

Patients may have legitimate concerns about the therapist. For instance, a patient who was sexually abused by a man may be uncomfortable in the presence of a male therapist. The patient may be concerned about discussing issues of sexuality and other issues that might be embarrassing or even prohibited by religion or cultural expectations. Patients generally want to be seen by someone who understands their specific experience or perspective. For example, a transgender patient may be interested in being seen by an LGBTQ therapist or gender- or sexuality-affirming therapist. In addition, while research evidence indicates that matching patients and therapists on demographic characteristics does not impact treatment outcome (Barkham

& Lambert, 2021), there are situations where matching therapists is desirable and important. Therapists and administrators should be responsive to such requests. With the recent advent of trauma-informed perspectives and increased awareness of structural prejudices, patients may be more likely to want to be treated by someone who shares demographic characteristics or life experiences. These kinds of requests need to be fully considered, openly discussed, and respected when possible.

At times, concerns about the therapist may reflect the patient's psychological concerns and difficulties in trusting the therapist. For example, an intake meeting was conducted with a woman who had been sexually abused by her father. The therapist was male, and the patient belonged to a different cultural group from the therapist, although this cultural difference was not immediately apparent. When discussing the patient at an intake meeting, the therapist raised the possibility of continuing with the patient in therapy after the evaluation. Another clinician objected to the patient being treated by a male therapist and advocated for the patient to be seen by a female therapist, given her sexual abuse history. Further concerns were raised about the cultural differences between the therapist and patient, and this was highlighted as a potential barrier to treatment. The therapist who conducted the intake assessment did not perceive any tension or difficulty during the intake. Such concerns related to a male therapist in this situation are understandable, while at the same time, there is a chance that a male therapist may foster corrective relationship experiences. When the patient was asked about her preference, she indicated that she preferred to be seen by the male therapist.

It is important to avoid being dismissive or defensive in response to a patient's questions or concerns. A therapist's failure to respond directly to a patient's questions can be easily and mistakenly justified by concerns about self-disclosure and boundaries. Self-disclosure is discouraged more in specific psychodynamic therapies (i.e., transference-focused psychotherapy) than in other approaches, given the emphasis on therapeutic neutrality. The rationale for therapist neutrality stems from the aim of not unduly influencing the patient's perspective with therapist content. However, maintaining neutrality with patients with disorders who can exhibit high levels of mistrust can run the risk of furthering mistrust. A way to respond to questions by the patient is to be open and willing to answer them while being curious about what may underlie the questions. Acknowledging that questions will be answered can reduce mistrust.

At times, therapists will encounter patients who express prejudicial ideas. Some therapists maintain that it is the role of the therapist to tolerate such comments while engaging the patient therapeutically. These are personal decisions that can be discussed with colleagues and supervisors. Nonetheless, it can be helpful to address these issues psychologically and through a social justice lens. Prejudicial comments can arise in response to a patient's defensiveness, concerns about trust, and worries about gaining support. When handled therapeutically, the therapist can promote the therapeutic alliance and the treatment process. To illustrate, consider the following dilemma faced by the Austrian–Chilean psychiatrist Otto Kernberg, who, as a child, escaped Nazi persecution and, years later, while living in Chile, treated the son of a prominent Nazi who escaped prosecution by fleeing to South America (personal communication, April 7, 2023). Kernberg fled Vienna at the age of 10 in the middle of the night with one suitcase just as the Nazis entered Austria. Much of his family perished in the Holocaust. When asked how he could treat such a person, his response was twofold. First, he thought he could help the patient be a better person if he treated him. Second, he recognized that the patient had been mistreated in his own family in a manner similar to how the Nazis treated Jewish people. Thus, he could identify an avenue for sympathy.

Recognizing the psychological dynamics underlying such utterances in therapy can help the therapist respond therapeutically. Therapists might find themselves saying things such as, "Sounds like, with our differences, it is difficult for you to imagine that someone like me could be helpful to you," or simply, "It is hard to know if you can trust me." Allowing for the discussion of such topics often creates a kind of trust that would otherwise be difficult to build.

What should the therapist do if the patient criticizes the therapy task or methods proposed by the therapist?

Consider the following scenario: A patient who was referred to a dialectical behavior therapy (DBT) therapist stated, "I have already done DBT. Is that what you are proposing to me again? DBT has not helped me." Several responses may be considered in this scenario. Firstly, it may be true that previous therapy (i.e., DBT) was unhelpful, although there are many reasons for such unhelpfulness that are unrelated to the actual therapy approach. A possible helpful move would be to validate the patient's disappointment about the failure of previous treatments to reach their goals and explore the factors that contributed to the poor outcome. Second, if the patient directly asked whether there is another technique or approach for the treatment of their difficulties, the therapist may want to provide information about other treatments (if the diagnosis of personality disorder had already been confirmed)— for example, "You mentioned there might be other therapy approaches for treating personality disorders. Yes, there are a few others I can recommend to you, including [name them]. I can offer you a few names of colleagues who have been trained in these approaches." Providing direct, clear, and accurate information to the patient is not only respectful but can also help increase the patient's sense of trust in the relationship. Finally, if the patient's diagnosis is still unclear, it may be important to assess the patient's goals and problems before recommending any specific approach.

What should the therapist do if the patient criticizes therapy in general, including experiences with past therapists and concurrent treatments?

Not infrequently, patients enter a first session feeling skeptical about treatment. For example, one patient stated, "I really don't like therapy. Therapists are only nice to patients so they can take money from honest people, and I don't have much money. I am here because I was referred. But I really hate therapy, and I always get worse with therapy." This overgeneralized and critical statement can be challenging. Psychotherapists often assume that patients enter into treatment motivated to receive help. However, therapists may realize quickly that motivation is a problem for many patients with personality disorders and is not a prerequisite to treatment. It can be helpful to acknowledge and validate the difficulty expressed by the patient—for example, "It must be hard for you to be here today, given that you say you hate therapy. I wonder what I can do to make this experience less negative and more bearable for you." Next, the therapist can unpack the patient's remark—for example, "What does it mean to 'hate' therapy?" How did the patient come to the conclusion that all therapists want is to take money "from honest citizens" (implicitly and sweepingly accusing the psychotherapy professions of dishonesty)? Exploring the patient's comment is imperative to addressing the barriers to engagement. It could be that the patient never received effective psychotherapy for their difficulties, and this needs to be clarified.

Managing Suicidal, Self-Harming, and Impulsive Behaviors

What should the therapist do if the patient arrives at the first session under the influence of alcohol or drugs?

This is, unfortunately, not an uncommon scenario. Consider the following situation with a patient who presented at the first session under the influence of alcohol. This may be apparent to the therapist shortly into a virtual session when the patient starts slurring his words and appears to nod off. When behaviors interfering with therapy arise in session, they need to be addressed directly with the patient. Failure to address such issues directly may give an unhelpful message that any behavior is tolerable, and this interferes with a constructive therapy process down the road. The therapist may respond by saying, "It seems to me that you are having a hard time focusing on our conversation right now. You said that you had a few drinks before you came in today. Is that right?" The therapist may continue, "You know, I want to make sure that you get the most out of your therapy sessions. So, it is important for me to tell you that you should come in sober next time. Can we agree on this?" If the patient is too intoxicated and unable to process information, it may be necessary to terminate the session early. It is important to discuss limits related to problematic behaviors that interfere with therapy to protect the therapeutic space and increase collaboration in the therapeutic process. Some therapists may be afraid to discuss these issues explicitly; however, it is usually necessary and critical to effective therapy.

What should the therapist do if the patient speaks of self-harming and suicidal urges in the first session?

Patients may present to session communicating self-harming or suicidal urges. This is a quick start to therapy. For some patients, it may also be a way to communicate the desperation of the situation and the desire for help. The therapist may respond by reinforcing the patient for seeking help and attending the session. For example, the therapist could say, "It is so good you are here. I'd really like to understand what you're struggling with. I imagine there is something underlying these urges that must be overwhelming. Can we look at what is going on that is leading you to think about self-harm right now?" Within the framework of DBT, this exploration entails an assessment of various influencing factors, such as triggers in interpersonal relationships, environmental vulnerabilities (e.g., lack of support or structure), and the associated emotions and thoughts propelling the urges. Depending on the effectiveness of this process, the therapist can then discuss with the patient what proved helpful, saying, for instance, "It seems like you're finding it easier to manage your urges now. What do you think contributed to this positive outcome today?"

What should the therapist do if the patient makes strong threats to commit suicide at the end of the first session?

Threats of suicide by a patient should always be taken seriously. The therapist should avoid panicking and focus on assessing the real risk. For some patients, expressions of suicide are a chronic and habitual pattern of thinking and may not be associated with imminent risk of suicide. The therapist should seek to understand the patient's current suicide communication in the context of their history of suicidal behavior. It is important to assess whether the factors controlling the current suicidal communication are linked to past high-risk suicidal behaviors. Does the patient have a viable plan, an intent to act on the plan, and a means to act on the plan? What is the risk associated with the proposed plan? On the basis of an assessment of suicide risk, the therapist can decide how to intervene. It is always advisable to seek consultation with a supervisor or senior colleague who is experienced in suicide risk assessments.

Depending on the suicide risk, the therapist may implement a range of interventions, such as additional telephone contact, additional sessions within working hours, emergency room visits, or hospitalization in a psychiatric unit. Preferably, decisions about the treatment plan and management of suicide should be made collaboratively with the patient. The advantages and drawbacks of each intervention should be considered, including the discussion of commitment and contracts to not engage in these behaviors. Minimizing the real risk of death in the short and long term is the goal. It is not helpful to respond in an anxious manner and become overly active in trying to rescue a patient because it is counterproductive to increasing the patient's active coping. A low-intensity interaction that focuses on increasing the patient's level of active problem solving is preferable in these situations.

Establishing a Treatment Frame

What should the therapist do if the patient does not show up for the first session?

When a patient does not show up for a first session, it can be a tricky situation to navigate because the therapist has little knowledge about the patient to act on. The therapist's response will depend on several contextual aspects. For example, it depends on whether there has been previous telephone contact between the therapist and patient and whether the therapist has information from other sources about the patient so far (e.g., a referral letter discussing an acute danger of suicide or self-harm). First, the therapist is advised to wait and not panic because many patients in need of treatment call back in these situations. Then, with the available information, the therapist or the person who took the appointment for them may want to contact the patient and inquire about possible misunderstandings related to the scheduled and missed meeting. It is important to point out that sometimes-repeated outreaches through different channels (i.e., email, voice mail, letter) may be necessary to encourage the patient to attend an appointment.

What should the therapist do if the patient says they do not want to be there but has presented to treatment under pressure by a third party (e.g., an intimate partner)?

During the first session, while the therapist is exploring the reasons for seeking therapy, it may become clear the patient does not want to be in treatment and showed up because of pressure from a third party. An intimate partner may have threatened to end the relationship if the patient does not go to therapy. Under the pressure of interpersonal loss, many people may comply and consult a therapist. However, in these situations, the motivation of the patient can be low, and this can be a challenge. In the first session, the therapeutic task is not to develop a stringent treatment focus but to enhance motivation and engagement. This usually requires warmly welcoming the patient, recognizing collaboratively that "we have a problem here," and constructing a positive working atmosphere. The therapist can acknowledge the odd feeling of being in a situation where the patient does not want to be there. The therapist may say, "It must be odd to sit here and speak to me when you don't want to be here and when you're thinking that your partner is the one who should be in therapy. How is it for you to be here right now?" The therapist can explore why the patient's partner thinks the patient needs therapy. Aligning with the patient's confusion, the therapist could express surprise or slight confusion as to why someone may think that way and, at the same time, be open to any new relevant information about the patient's behavior (in the eyes of both the patient and, presumably, the partner).

What should the therapist do if the patient says they "only" want psychopharmacotherapy?

In clinical situations in which a patient insists that medication is the only solution to their problems, the therapist may adopt a cautious and open attitude because, in the first session, it is impossible to have a comprehensive picture of the patient and presenting problems and treatment options. If the patient insists that medications are a condition for further therapy (which is seldom the case, in our experience), the therapist can explore the problem that medications will be used to treat. The therapist may review the patient's medication history, including the usefulness of specific medications and side effects, to understand the patient's perspective on the role of medication (this may also be done with the help of a pharmacologist). This information may help the therapist better understand the role of medications in treatment while at the same time grasp a sense of the patient's perceived core problems. Should a personality disorder diagnosis be confirmed, the therapist may explain that medication will not cure these problems but will, at best, only partially attenuate certain symptom clusters (and, in addition, create undesirable side effects). Psychoeducation on biological determinants of behaviors and the biological effects of psychotherapy may be helpful in some cases. Psychotherapy will help tackle the fundamental problems related to interpersonal relationships and emotional dysregulation pertaining to personality disorders.

What should the therapist do if the patient asks the therapist for their personal telephone number during the first session of therapy?

When a patient asks for the therapist's personal telephone number in the first session, it is a good opportunity for the therapist to discuss intersession contact. Therapists working with suicidal patients (e.g., certain patients with BPD) should provide a system of crisis coverage outside of the therapy hour. Depending on the psychotherapy approach, the context of the clinic where the therapist is working, and insurance coverage, therapists may be available to answer the patient's calls (e.g., during certain times; during general office hours, such as in DBT; by using a pager system around the clock). In certain approaches (i.e., DBT programs), it may be within the therapist's limits to provide a personal phone number to patients. For additional coverage, the therapist may inform the patient about alternative options, such as psychiatric emergency services, psychological helplines, and so forth. In the unlikely case that the patient insists that they need to call the therapist and no one else, the therapist can discuss their personal limits. From our experience, requests for out-of-session contact are rare. Most patients feel reassured if they understand where and whom to call in case of emergencies outside of appointments.

What should the therapist do if the patient is already receiving other psychotherapies?

Patients may report that they are already engaged in other treatments, including psychotherapy. In this case, the therapist may use the orientation sessions to clarify what, if anything, the current therapy could add to the overall treatment plan. It may make sense for the clinician to leave this question completely open at first contact. Often, patients may struggle with ending relationships with other therapy providers even when those treatments are not helpful. Time may be needed to help the patient gently end another therapy relationship. A detailed understanding of the role of different providers is needed to determine whether the overall treatment plan makes sense. It may be that supplementary treatments are not only unnecessary but also iatrogenic; in the case of multiple treatments, there may be interference of the effects and a lack of clarity regarding the helpfulness of a specific intervention. If a decision is made to offer multiple treatments with different providers, a meeting with the patient and other treatment providers is recommended to clarify roles and responsibilities.

CONCLUSIONS

In conclusion, beginning therapy with patients with personality disorders can be fraught with many challenges, some of which we discussed in this chapter. Many patients who schedule appointments for therapy do not show up for the first session, and many other patients drop out after the first few appointments. These risks of dropout are higher for patients with personality disorders than those without personality disorders (Swift & Greenberg, 2012; Wierzbicki & Pekarik, 1993). Among patients with personality disorders, the risk of early dropout is especially pronounced for those with BPD (Waldinger & Gunderson, 1987; Yeomans et al., 1994) and narcissistic personality disorder (Ellison et al., 2013; Hilsenroth et al., 1998).

Despite the challenges of treating patients with personality disorders, limited specialist training is typically provided to trainees (Levy & Ellison, 2022; Sansone et al., 2013). Little is known about how to train clinicians effectively to work with individuals with personality disorders. Some pre–post evaluations of workshop attendees have indicated that training reduces stigma and increases confidence in working with patients with personality disorders (Keuroghlian et al., 2016; Krawitz, 2004, Shanks et al., 2011). There are several reports on how to implement training on personality disorders in clinical psychology department clinics (Noll et al., 2020; Rizvi et al., 2017) and psychiatric residency programs (e.g., Bernstein et al., 2015; Unruh & Gunderson, 2016; Zerbo et al., 2013). However, there is scant research on the effectiveness of training programs.

Research is needed on how to develop basic competencies in treating individuals with personality disorders. First sessions are particularly important when working with individuals with personality disorders. Therapists need to be skilled in facilitating patient engagement, establishing a clear treatment frame, and cultivating an effective relationship for therapy to be successful. More research is needed to determine how therapists can effectively engage patients early in treatment (Culina et al., 2022). Effectively balancing relational and technical skills is especially important. Future work should focus on training therapist skills. We suggest that deliberate practice—the intentional repetition of helping skills, using tailored feedback from video-recorded or live sessions in psychotherapy training—is a useful approach to train therapists across a range of challenging clinical scenarios to improve specific skills to enhance abilities to respond effectively.

4 MOVING FROM EMOTIONAL DYSREGULATION TO EMOTIONAL BALANCE

This chapter explores changes in the functional domain of emotional dysregulation in patients with personality pathology on the premise that such changes are responsible for the effects of treatment. We first consider broad empirical support for the role of change in emotional dysregulation in the treatment of personality pathology. We then present the case of Marcus, a patient whose treatment and subsequent recovery were marked by a concentration on emotional regulation.[1] Our case discussion focuses on the therapist's engagement with Marcus's apparent experience of shame and the more core emotional experiences underlying it. We next examine how the inappropriate expression of emotions can be addressed and how therapists can foster a greater emotional balance that is underpinned by higher levels of emotional awareness and regulation. These approaches are especially indicated to prevent dysregulated states and impulsive behavior, which are common in patients with borderline pathology. We end the chapter with a summary statement on how change in emotional dysregulation can be understood as a mechanism of change.

---

[1]The case of Marcus has been modified to disguise the patient's identity and protect his confidentiality.

https://doi.org/10.1037/0000388-005
Understanding Mechanisms of Change in Psychotherapies for Personality Disorders, by U. Kramer, K. N. Levy, and S. McMain

EMPIRICAL SUPPORT FOR CHANGE IN EMOTIONAL DYSREGULATION AS A MECHANISM OF CHANGE

Of the five mechanisms that have been identified as possible processes of change for the treatment of personality disorders, empirical support for change in the functional domain of emotional dysregulation is by far the most robust, despite it too being tentative. In Chapter 2, we established that emotional dysregulation plays a role in personality disorder patients' experiences of negative affect on a moment-by-moment and day-by-day basis and that there are consistent neurobiological underpinnings for this dysregulation (related to impaired modulatory function of the prefrontal cortices of the limbic system), especially in the face of interpersonally relevant negative stimuli. Change in emotional dysregulation is, therefore, a strong candidate for explaining psychotherapy outcomes for patients with personality disorders, borderline personality disorder (BPD) in particular. Change in emotional dysregulation may manifest both directly in the furtherment of emotional regulation and indirectly through (a) increased depth of emotional processing, (b) greater emotional awareness, and (c) emotional transformation.

Greater capacity for emotion regulation is particularly seen as core to progress in dialectical behavior therapy (DBT; Linehan et al., 2007). A literature review analyzed the mechanisms of change for BPD in both DBT and cognitive behavior therapy (CBT; Rudge et al., 2020) and concluded that insofar as these treatments are effective, the effect occurs through patients' uptake of more effective emotion regulation skills in daily life. One of the studies included in that review, McMain et al. (2013), showed specifically that in both DBT and good psychiatric management (GPM), emotional balance—conceptualized here as the patient's capacity to counterbalance positive and negative affect—predicted a decrease in symptoms above all other variables.

Although not all studies have as clearly identified emotion regulation as a mechanism of change in treatments for personality disorders, those that have not still consistently leave room for the possibility of an additional, conceivably more fundamental mechanism of change beyond the ones proposed. Another study included in the review by Rudge et al. (2020) was a mediation analysis by Neacsiu, Rizvi, and Linehan (2010) on change in self-reported skills uptake (the proposed mechanism of change in most theories of DBT) in patients with BPD. These authors found that while skills uptake mediated the decrease in self-harm behaviors, it did not mediate more specific emotion-related outcomes, such as anger suppression and expression. This suggests that there is another mechanism of change at play in these emotion-related outcomes: quite possibly, the emotional balance as identified by McMain et al. (2013).

The third study included in the review was that of Kramer, Pascual-Leone, Berthoud, et al. (2016), which assessed changes in anger as a potential mechanism of change. While changes in anger were indeed seen in symptomatically improved groups, these authors identified the specific changes as increased "assertive anger"—the expression of anger that was functionally related to adaptive needs for boundary setting and identity—which may more broadly be understood as a form of emotion regulation. In a secondary analysis of this same study, Kramer (2017) assessed emotion regulation skills directly as they were observed in-session in standardized pre- and post-research interviews alongside the DBT skills training component. This study showed an increase in productive in-session coping skills (and a decrease in unproductive coping skills) in DBT only, which were associated with changes in outcomes (compared with a waitlist control). The effects of "productive coping," as described by Kramer (2017), also align with what is understood elsewhere as emotion regulation. As such, there is at least an indication that emotion regulation is involved, even with proposed mechanisms of change that, on the face of it, do not appear related. In DBT especially, but also across diverse treatment methods, including CBT and GPM, emotion regulation recurs as either an explicitly or implicitly related factor in recovery.

Uptake of more productive emotion regulation skills may be central for BPD patients undergoing any treatment, not only DBT. In a mediation analysis of a brief version of GPM, Kramer et al. (2017) looked at reductions in in-session behavioral coping strategies, which are described as impulsive behaviors to regulate tension, such as acting out. Such behaviors indicate poor emotion regulation, and the goal is to minimize them. The authors observed that a decrease in behavioral coping strategies between Sessions 1 and 5 mediated a relief in symptoms between Sessions 5 and 10. Again, these decreases and the corresponding symptomatic relief may be explained by improved emotion regulation.

A more recent study, again using mediation analysis on a sample of patients with BPD undergoing DBT skills training compared with a waitlist control, tested whether distress tolerance and mindfulness are potential mechanisms of change explaining outcomes (Zeifman et al., 2020). The findings showed that the outcomes were explained both by improvements in mindfulness capacities and the increased applications of distress tolerance techniques. Mindfulness and distress tolerance both constitute specific functions of emotion regulation, further supporting the notion of emotion regulation as a mechanism of change in treatments of personality pathology.

Enhanced emotion regulation is also associated with the neurofunctional changes in patients with BPD seen across different psychotherapies. In a meta-analysis, Marceau et al. (2018) analyzed studies showing neurobiological changes between pre- and posttreatment of patients with BPD and found a consistent picture with the psychologically anchored findings described previously: Brain regions that are associated with executive control and emotion regulation were enhanced after treatment. A number of smaller studies (Driessen et al., 2009; Perez et al., 2016; Schnell & Herpertz, 2007) found at the end of treatment altered functioning (i.e., back toward a healthy normal) in neuronal regions known to be involved in increased effectiveness of emotion regulation. These regions involve, among others, the amygdala, the left anterior insula, the anterior cingulate gyrus, the precuneus, and the hippocampus. In a large, well-controlled study, Schmitt et al. (2016) found increased functional connectivity between the orbitofrontal cortex, subgenual anterior cingulate cortex, dorsolateral prefrontal cortex, and the insula and amygdala—a network of regions responsible for the modulation of emotion. These results underscore the role of biological substrates in the increased effectiveness of emotion regulation as a potential mechanism of change in therapy for BPD.

Alternative conceptual lenses have been adopted to define change in emotional dysregulation with regard to depth of emotional processing, emotion awareness (e.g., Lane et al., 2022), and emotion transformation. Transformation in emotion may follow a moment-by-moment sequential pattern from less differentiated global distress due to poorly identified and expressed experiences of specific emotions, such as fear or shame or loneliness, to well-differentiated emotion awareness and resolution (e.g., by accessing healthy anger; Pascual-Leone, 2018). The latter has been studied in greater detail in emotion-focused therapy. This change in differentiation has been tested both within-session and between-session for explaining outcomes across samples with personality disorders. For BPD specifically, two studies have examined change in emotional processing from this theoretical viewpoint. In addition to the study by Kramer, Pascual-Leone, Berthoud, et al. (2016) discussed previously, Berthoud et al. (2017) showed a decrease in the frequency of in-session global distress (i.e., an undifferentiated, sometimes ill-regulated emotion state) over the course of psychiatric treatment, which was believed to partially explain the decrease in interpersonal problems.

For patients with other personality disorders (mostly narcissistic and histrionic) undergoing a form of client-centered psychotherapy (i.e., with a focus on proactive clarification), Kramer, Pascual-Leone, Rohde, et al. (2016) showed that the expression of anger, as well as in-session access to self-compassionate emotions, explain good symptom evolution. Expression of anger (again, healthy, assertive anger styles) reflects strengthened emotion regulation, as does an enhanced ability to self-regulate through self-compassionate emotion. For the subsample with narcissistic personality disorder, Kramer, Pascual-Leone, et al. (2018) found that when patients were speaking about topics related to the self, small decreases in in-session access to and expression of shame were predictive of symptom decrease and explained a more compassionate stance toward the self later in treatment. As such, regulating shame experiences, which can be diffuse and overwhelming in personality-disordered patients, appears to be core to the functionality of emotion regulation in symptom improvement.

In the next section, we turn our attention to the case study.

THE CASE OF MARCUS

Marcus is a 28-year-old man who self-identifies as male and heterosexual. He has a PhD in mathematics and holds a postdoctorate position at a university lab. A recent breakup with his girlfriend, Laura, with whom he lived for 3 years, left him reeling and feeling abandoned, and he is not currently in another relationship. He reported that he had been in a depressive and anxious mood throughout the 5 months before the breakup, with incidences of irritation, impulsivity, and angry outbursts. This led to Laura stating that if he did not consult a psychotherapist, she would end their relationship. He also reported difficulties in concentrating on his work, feelings of emptiness, and a sense of absence of direction in his life. After the breakup, these symptoms worsened, and he started to self-harm by cutting his forearms when feeling distressed and lonely, and he developed repetitive suicidal thoughts. He reported that he had engaged in heavy binge drinking and regular cannabis consumption up to 1 year earlier but had managed to control this thanks to specialist consultation.

Marcus presented with BPD and dysthymia. From a dimensional viewpoint (*Diagnostic and Statistical Manual of Mental Disorders* [5th ed., text rev.] alternative model five trait domains; American Psychiatric Association, 2022), he presented high on negative affectivity, detachment, and disinhibition, and low on antagonism and psychoticism.

The patient reported having a distant relationship with his father but a rather close one with his mother. He described his father as a workaholic who was never present for him when he was a child and did not open up to him on important issues. This left him feeling alone and seeking support only from his mother, whom he portrayed as a warm person with whom he felt comfortable discussing all kinds of issues and problems—for example, being bullied at school for several months when he was 11 years old. He has a few close male friends but said that he had neglected them over the past few months, concentrating almost exclusively on his relationship with Laura. He said that he is successful in his work and is generally seen as likable by his colleagues.

Marcus was initially reluctant to fully engage in treatment but eventually became motivated, stating, a bit anxiously, that he wanted to overcome his problems as quickly as possible. He built some trust with the therapist and then engaged in therapy fairly easily. He readily reported any self-harming behaviors and suicidal thoughts he experienced but expressed shame about them. He mentioned that he felt embarrassed about his self-destructive tendencies and wished to hide them from others, including the therapist.

The therapist felt that Marcus's difficulties with emotion regulation might explain his self-harming behaviors and other emotional difficulties (sadness, loneliness, feelings of rejection, irritation, and anger), and Marcus agreed to work on this from a DBT perspective.

CASE FORMULATION: UNDERSTANDING THE CORE EMOTION DISTURBANCE

Case formulation is the basis for providing meaning to multilayered and often ambiguous information and may offer a framework for intervention (Eells, 2022). We begin by considering how to conceptualize Marcus's apparent emotional problems and how they manifest in therapy.

A host of emotions are at the forefront of Marcus's case, among which are sadness, shame, and anger. Shame is one of the core emotion disturbances: Marcus expressed shame and embarrassment in the therapeutic relationship, which he described directly and which also manifested on the level of nonverbal behavior (e.g., hesitancies in the narrative and repeatedly looking down at the floor when trying to respond to the therapist's prompts and questions). When describing behaviors or experiences that led to his self-harming in particular situations, he used descriptions such as "so embarrassing" and "so shameful." It is clear that shame is a central component of Marcus's case, but what role it plays in his symptomatology, treatment trajectory, and outcome needs to be further assessed.

Twice in the vignette, the patient mentioned feeling shame: The first was after engaging in a parasuicidal behavior, and the second was when he described feeling heavy, empty, and ashamed, and then hating himself (which may also be understood as shame) as a precipitant of self-destructive behaviors. The latter is different from the shame expressed after such behaviors. There is also the question of whether the patient's initial reluctance to engage in therapy is a behavior due to shame (which may be a secondary experience to more primary emotions). Alternatively, it could be reluctance due to paranoia and/or feeling unsure of what the experience would be like. There are many different ways to understand the patient's shame and its role and context in his symptomatic presentation and treatment response. The role of case formulation is to examine under multiple lenses each possibility for working toward a cohesive, rich, and precise understanding.

Dialectical Behavior Formulation: Five Steps to an Individualized Formation

The implementation of DBT is guided by an individualized case formulation. One fundamental assumption underlying this formulation is that pervasive emotional dysregulation problems are the foundation for personality pathology. Symptoms, in this context, either function as a means to regulate distressing emotions or arise as a consequence of dysregulated emotions.

Constructing a highly individualized formulation involves four key steps. First, the therapist assesses the patient's problems and gathers information about the factors contributing to and maintaining their difficulties and symptoms. This includes evaluating the range, severity, and duration of the patient's problems, symptoms, and coexisting disorders and identifying specific emotional dysregulation deficits. This information helps determine the patient's level of severity, stage of treatment, and appropriate treatment focus. For individuals with severe behavioral dyscontrol problems, the initial stage of treatment centers on enhancing stability. The formulation incorporates the patient's treatment goals and primary targets, with the session focus guided by a hierarchical consideration. High-priority targets related to life-threatening, treatment-interfering, and quality-of-life impairing issues take precedence over lower priority targets. In addition, the therapist assesses microlevel expressions of problematic patterns of emotional dysregulation, such as extreme shifts in emotional modulation, the expression of emotional needs, and the tolerance of aversive primary emotions. Last, the therapist explores the patient's developmental history, paying attention to biological and environmental factors that contributed to their emotional dysregulation problems. The current environmental situation is also evaluated because it influences the maintenance of difficulties and may impact treatment progress.

Second, in collaboration with the patient, the therapist conducts behavioral chain analyses to uncover the unique factors controlling specific behaviors. This includes identifying vulnerability factors, typical triggers, emotions and cognitions, actions, and consequences associated with particular responses. The identified controlling factors inform decisions regarding which behaviors need modification or reinforcement.

Third, the therapist compares data from multiple chain analyses to identify recurring problematic patterns and determine areas of focus.

Fourth, the therapist uses the information gathered from the macro- and microlevel assessment to determine the intervention focus and select appropriate interventions.

Finally, in the fifth step, an intervention plan is developed. By summarizing information from multiple chain analyses and recognizing patterns across behaviors, minitreatment plans are constructed, tested, and revised according to the patient's response.

On the basis of the description of Marcus, it is evident that he struggles with effectively regulating intense emotions and tolerating emotional distress. He has a history of anger outbursts, self-harm, and substance abuse, which likely serve as coping mechanisms to escape overwhelming internal aversive emotions. Marcus also exhibits high levels of self-criticism, potentially as a cognitive strategy to evade overwhelming emotional experiences. He perceives himself as likable yet reports having few friends and avoiding relationships with men, suggesting avoidance behaviors to protect himself from anticipated aversive emotions associated with criticism and rejection. Given his significant self-loathing, shame appears to be a primary maladaptive emotion, although it may also arise as a secondary emotion due to self-criticism. Marcus's description of his emotionally distant and unavailable father and his history of being bullied provides a historical context for the invalidating experiences that contributed to his development of emotion regulation problems.

The implications of this formulation for intervention are twofold. First, it will be crucial to enhance Marcus's awareness and tolerance of underlying primary emotions. Simultaneously, it will be important to help him develop alternative strategies to delay impulsive urges aimed at escaping overwhelming emotions. Engaging Marcus in a behavioral chain analysis of specific instances of his problematic behaviors, such as self-harm, is suggested as a means to increase his insight into the factors controlling these behaviors.

Transference-Focused Formulation: An Object Relations Perspective

Transference-focused formulation derives from Kernberg's (1984) object relations theory. As such, information for the formulation is drawn from three sources (Levy et al., 2019): (a) the assessment of clinical symptoms, (b) the assessment of the intrapsychic structure and functioning, and (c) the assessment of the quality of the therapeutic relationship. To do so, the therapist takes into account verbal and nonverbal communication, as well as the therapist's countertransferential reactions. The case formulation is based on what Kernberg (1984) called the structural interview, which is designed to assess the patient's psychological structure. During the structural interview, the therapist assesses the patient's mental status, obtains a complete symptom picture to make differential diagnoses, assesses the patient's current level of functioning, and probes the patient's sense of self and others. Toward the end of the interview, the therapist may begin to assess how the patient responds to a psychotherapeutic technique called trial interpretation.

The information is used to establish the patient's level of personality organization and personality style and provide the patient with feedback regarding the therapist's initial formulations of the patient's problems. This information is used to collaboratively establish the treatment frame and assess the patient's willingness to engage in treatment. The construction of the structural interview is hierarchical or cyclical, which means that certain items need to be prioritized, and the patient's answers to each step determine the content of the formulation. First, the therapist asks for presenting problems (e.g., symptoms, relationships), then moves to pathological personality traits, then to identity and reality testing. This latter triad helps determine the presence of a borderline condition in the patient and is the core of the assessment of personality disorders. In addition, further steps involve the assessment of functional psychosis (on the levels of behavior, affect, thought, and florid positive psychotic symptoms) and organic brain syndromes (including functions related to the sensorium, memory, and intelligence). This information is integrated with the information from the countertransferential reactions, and the synthesis of this transference-focused formulation will then be used in an experience-near language in communication with the patient. It appears that the transference-focused formulation is particularly adapted for patients diagnosed with personality disorders and who have problems with identity and interpersonal antagonism. From a relationship viewpoint, the transference-focused formulation is an opportunity to convey a deep understanding of all aspects of the patient's experience, which is typically done using timely interpretations.

From a transference-focused psychotherapy (TFP) perspective (Yeomans et al., 2015), what is more central for Marcus than shame is self-criticism, although, obviously, shame can be linked with self-criticism. Experiences of criticism are integral to any TFP formulation: One can be critical or hard about or on oneself and can also experience others being critical about or hard on oneself. Likewise, one can be critical of others. For patients with BPD, it is especially important to ask who is being hard on whom. Clarity on the source of the experience of criticism can be elusive in BPD because the boundaries between self and other can be blurred due to identity disturbance, producing misunderstandings about the source of criticism as internal versus external.

Marcus's initial reluctance to start therapy may be in part due to shame in talking about the difficult behaviors he has engaged in. He might feel embarrassed or ashamed about honest disclosure, and these feelings are amplified when he thinks the other person is viewing him negatively or with judgment. He is critical of himself—ashamed on his own account—but also thinks the other person might be critical, judging or evaluating him or seeing him negatively. As a result, upon the initiation of treatment, he was reluctant to share. However, as he built trust with the therapist, he was able to share more openly. We can infer that as Marcus's trust in his therapist and willingness to disclose increase, his feelings of self-criticism and expectation of others' judgment recede into the background. Marcus's increased capacity for disclosure also tracks improved self-awareness and regulation of his sense of self and others. As in DBT, TFP aims to understand the feelings of shame and associated behaviors as "escape behaviors" (see the previous section). While shame may be apparent, we need to understand this emotion in the context of the self-critical position the patient adopts toward himself. This contextualization of shame as a feeling resulting from self-criticism and the expectation of others' criticism opens avenues of intervention, and the symptomatology, including shame, may be resolvable by working with Marcus on his experience of criticism from self and others and reconciling his internal views of himself.

Plan Analysis Formulation: Synthesizing Integrative Therapy With Motivation Science

Plan analysis as a case formulation method builds on the framework of integrative psychological therapy developed by Grawe (1998) and Caspar (2019, 2022) focusing on individualizing the treatment to each patient with concepts from motivation science. In contrast with other case formulation methods that draw directly from specific psychotherapy models, plan analysis stands on its own ground as a theory-independent methodology to individualized case formulations, which may thus be understood as a means of psychotherapy integration. The formulation is done by the therapist according to clinical material from the patient (verbal, paraverbal, and nonverbal aspects of communication), as well as the therapist's reactions and action tendencies toward a particular patient in a particular situation. In the formulation, observable behaviors and experiences are differentiated from instrumentally linked behavior underlying plans and motives. The latter is part of the hypothesized internal determinants explaining the presenting problems and resources of the patient.

A plan analysis is typically depicted on paper where the instrumental links between behaviors (and experiences, as a means to an end), plans, and motives (or goals) become evident. Plans may be defined according to possible instrumentality with behaviors, answering the question of what purposes serve specific behaviors and experiences. A patient's plan analysis helps the therapist conceptualize and anticipate potential interpersonal problems or stalemates in the therapeutic relationship and their resources and helps select the appropriate intervention for the presenting problem. Specifically, the motive-oriented therapeutic relationship may be constructed proactively according to the acceptable underlying motives established for a patient through plan analysis. It is assumed that a therapist who provides this type of relationship offers the patient a corrective emotional experience in the therapy hour because the problematic means to pursue acceptable goals become superfluous in the interaction. Research evidence tends to confirm these assumptions (Caspar, 2019, 2022; Kramer, 2020). Information from the plan analysis is, therefore, mostly used implicitly (on the relationship level) and is made explicit when needed with the patient. It appears that plan analysis is particularly appropriate for patients with personality disorders with problematic self-direction and typical antagonism in the relationship (Kramer, 2019).

From a plan analysis perspective (Caspar, 2019), Marcus's self-harming behaviors may be understood as being reactive to other emotions as a means of coping with more intense experiences he wants to avoid. Interestingly, these (and other coping behaviors) do not have the instrumental component seen in other clinical cases. There seems to be no direct interpersonal gain to Marcus from engaging in these behaviors, although the expression of secondary shame might serve the purpose of his being "treated with delicacy" as a result (e.g., in the therapeutic relationship). Without a clear instrumental component, the functional and controlling variables of Marcus's self-harming behaviors are strong candidates for a DBT approach.

The plan analysis perspective may also focus on the self-criticism component mentioned earlier: It may be related to difficulty with self-worth. Paradoxically, Marcus seems to use a whole host of escape behaviors—including impulsivity, outbursts, self-harming, and yelling at others—to maintain his self-image and his self-concept as a "good partner," to stay with Laura as long as possible, and to start therapy in an attempt to maintain the intimate relationship with her (even though he did not feel the need to come in the first place). Marcus's behaviors may function as a desperate attempt to externalize his feelings of self-doubt to avoid internally confronting them. In conclusion, from a plan analysis perspective, it appears that Marcus's self-harming behaviors may, in fact, be instrumental in the sense that they are coping behaviors serving higher level plans related to maintaining a positive self-image in interpersonal relationships.

This analysis does not deemphasize the role of emotion regulation; on the contrary, Marcus's coping behaviors are both forms of and responses to emotional dysregulation. Conversely, the development of self-worth should co-occur with an increase in his capacity to self-regulate emotion. Intervention may focus on increasing the effectiveness of emotion regulation, both as a terminal goal to replace dysfunctional coping behaviors and as an intermediary method of facilitating self-awareness and internally sourced self-worth.

Toward a Common Formulation

Despite different emphases across different formulation viewpoints, numerous common themes and points of collision appear. We tend to agree that, for Marcus, being around other people triggers distress and that an even greater trigger for him is the transition between being with others and being alone. Thus, he is emotionally activated by seeing his therapist and then leaving the session, socializing with friends and then going home, and having somebody contact him and then ending the conversation. This may, in part, be linked to his personal history of being bullied and having an emotionally unavailable father, and the impact of these invalidating experiences probably contributes to much of the underlying emotional pain. When triggered, he likely experiences some intolerable emotion, such as overwhelming loneliness, which is exacerbated as he alternates between having contact with others and having them leave. It is apparent that he experiences significant self-criticism, which likely generates secondary shame, and the shame, in turn, leads to self-harm and other escape behaviors. A secondary emotion here comes sequentially after a primary process (i.e., another emotion or a cognition). The self-perpetuating process probably goes something like this: "I tell myself that I'm no good, so then I feel lousy, so then I harm myself." There are also qualities of self-loathing and self-punishment that may contribute to the self-harming. Shame is clearly present, but all formulations concede that other emotions are even more primary and are likely generating the shame in a more complicated context. Shame may be seen as a secondary emotion, possibly a reactive experience to more core feelings, just as self-harm is a reactive experience to underlying emotional states.

Beyond the formulations we have seen and their common understanding of the patient's symptomatology as reactive, we can continue to ask at a deeper level, unlinked to any one methodology, which core emotional experiences are driving these reactive emotions and behaviors. To that question, there may be both problematic loneliness and core emptiness. These experiences may account for Marcus's difficulty tolerating being alone and remaining regulated when separating from others. Consequently, his coping behaviors, including self-harm, rumination, and yelling, may serve to avoid intense emotional experiences such as this loneliness or emptiness.

Interestingly, emptiness is something that Marcus explicitly talks about, and this sense of emptiness may be what leads him to feel abandoned when alone. This emptiness may make him fail to recognize what is inside him, be able to differentiate and identify emotions, or tolerate strong emotions. Most of us can use our representational world to understand, organize, and contextualize our experiences, like drops of water in the ocean, but for Marcus, transient individual experiences become the whole ocean. This patient has no means to metabolize or contextualize his experiences, and as a result, each one is overwhelming. This state of being overwhelmed is linked to emptiness insofar as the patient experiences having little within himself to serve as an anchor. This, too, is the link between emptiness and emotional dysregulation. In light of this, emptiness may be central to Marcus's case.

Emptiness, together with affect dysregulation, may be important in explaining self-harming behavior. Research has shown that emptiness may be an especially important construct in BPD (Miller et al., 2020). Emptiness may be seen as part of or at least related to identity disturbance. Clinical observation has revealed that people who are identity disturbed, if not diffused (see Chapter 6), often feel empty. Interestingly, this patient described something that, on the face of it, is contradictory: simultaneous heaviness and emptiness. Possibly, when he says "heaviness," he means feeling depressed or down. And when he says "empty," it is as if there is nothing to draw on. So, it makes sense, as we will see later, to teach him DBT skills, such as distress tolerance or interpersonal effectiveness, to help him recognize, identify, allow, tolerate, and then use effortful control to downregulate emotional reactions. These skills should both combat the depressive feelings and help provide an anchor for his feelings of having nothing to draw on. In addition, from a TFP perspective, the capacity to downregulate emotional reactions will facilitate increased identity integration, which in turn enables a greater capacity for regulating emotions.

From a research perspective, it has been shown that the affect dysregulation, such as self-loathing and shame, associated with self-injurious urges in BPD is a function of being in an identity-diffused state. In a study that used ecological momentary assessment to compare patients with BPD with patients with anxiety disorders, Scala et al. (2018) found a relationship between negative affect and urges to self-injure, moderated by whether the individual was in an identity-diffused state. In an identity-diffused state, one's self-concept is unclear. We can conclude that if you have a negative affect but a strong, cohesive sense of identity, you do not have the self-injurious urges associated with BPD. Only when you have a problematic self-concept do you experience those specific urges. From a different theoretical perspective, another study using ecological momentary assessment (Cardona et al., 2021) came to a consistent conclusion for a small sample of patients with BPD, showing that the level of intensity of BPD symptoms moderated the link between negative affectivity and self-harm. Yet another study found an association between chronic emptiness and the likelihood of suicide attempts (Grilo & Udo, 2021).

In conclusion, we agree that, while shame is present in Marcus's case, it does not represent the core maladaptive emotion, and the therapist needs to focus on that core emotion to help Marcus increase his emotional balance by accessing better emotion awareness and regulation. Either maladaptive loneliness or emptiness may be candidates for explaining the self-harming and other maladaptive behaviors apparent in this case (and which Marcus decided to focus on in his treatment). Focusing on core emptiness may have the advantage of encompassing both cognitive and affective components of the patient's experience and putting into greater context a cascade of events leading up to self-harming behavior (and other dysregulated affective experiences). In the case of Marcus, the increase of emotional awareness and effectiveness, whether by using newly learned skills or identifying and digging into the more core feelings underlying symptoms, is a primary goal of treatment. We see shame as more of a flare sent up by underlying issues that produce dysregulation, and we believe that as the dysregulation subsides, so will the shame.

CHOICE POINTS AND OPPORTUNITIES FOR CHANGE

For the remainder of this chapter, we present two choice points from the treatment offered to Marcus that were selected on the basis of the topics in the previous case formulation. The treatment followed a DBT approach, focusing globally on developing a more effective emotion regulation, in keeping with Marcus's main explicit motivation to decrease his self-harming and impulsive behaviors. First, we offer a summary of a chain analysis explicating self-harming behavior in a particular situation (from Session 5), then we recount a scene described by Marcus of a typical interaction with his then-girlfriend, Laura (from Session 10). At each juncture, we ask ourselves: What do we do here as psychotherapists? While parts of the content should focus on therapist interventions, we see each choice point as a unique opportunity for change in the patient by taking into consideration the mechanisms of change in psychotherapy. We end with a summary statement of gained knowledge and a discussion of research perspectives for mechanisms of change in treatments for patients with personality pathology, focusing on the change in emotional dysregulation. Table 4.1 synthesizes generic and approach-specific strategies that therapists might use, as well as relevant patient processes, in the two choice points presented in this chapter.

"I Just Had to Do It": Addressing the Emotional Precipitants of Self-Harming Behavior

In Session 5, Marcus described an incident from 2 days earlier of self-harming behavior:

> It was on Sunday. I was alone at home, nothing to do. I felt heavy inside, somewhat empty, I remember. I called a friend to see if he was around for stuff. He was with another friend, and they said I should come over to hang out with them. So I went. I had a good time in the afternoon with them, but that feeling inside of heaviness and emptiness never quite receded. So we had discussions about all kinds of things—girlfriends, soccer, and so on. Somehow, I felt a bit disconnected from the two and a bit tired all through the day. I decided to leave early to go to the gym, only to find out that the gym had already closed for the day. As I pushed open the door to my apartment, I had suicidal thoughts coming into my mind. It made me feel down, sad, and ashamed of myself.

TABLE 4.1. How to Foster a Path to Emotion Balance

Generic therapist interventions	Specific therapist interventions	Patient processes
Choice point: Addressing self-harming behavior		
• Do a case formulation.	• Do a chain analysis.	• Understand the precipitants.
• Offer acceptance in the relationship.	• Use validation strategies.	• Feel "normalized."
• Increase emotional awareness.	• Focus on underlying motives.	• Have a corrective experience.
• Modulate emotions and behaviors (e.g., teach distress tolerance).	• Avoid strengthening distortions.	• Be aware of distorted views.
• Teach interpersonal skills.	• Teach specific social support.	• Take up alternative skills.
		• Develop social resources.
Choice point: Addressing interpersonally dysregulated behavior with Laura		
• Do a case formulation.	• Do a chain analysis.	• Understand the precipitants.
• Assess precipitating events.	• Focus on emotion.	• Differentiate types of emotion.
• Foster interpersonal skills.	• Focus on self-criticism.	
	• Implement GIVE skills (be gentle, act interested, validate, and use an easy manner).	• Be aware of self-criticism.
• Foster emotion modulation.		• Learn to be gentle.

I hated myself at this moment so much! I found that I had no direction in my life, not knowing what really was important for me. This happens to me when I am alone. I felt the urge to cut, which I controlled for some time. I spent the evening playing piano, which helps to distract me. At 10 p.m., these urges became very strong, so I just had to do it. So I cut myself, just superficially, you know, but still. It was only a small injury, but I feel so ashamed about all this. It's so embarrassing.

This situation reveals the patient's difficulty in modulating his emotions effectively. According to our shared formulation, the statement about embarrassment and shame may represent a more secondary emotion, while emptiness or loneliness may be core to Marcus's experience. What would be needed here? What would be needed when he says, "I just had to do it"? Obviously, there is information to be gleaned from this excerpt through a chain analysis, as described later.

We now turn to what is needed in terms of therapist intervention, given our formulations and our understanding of this case so far. As noted in the Introduction, the following information is transcribed from actual dialogues held among us.

Dialectical Behavior Perspective: Validate the Urge

From a DBT perspective, an initial response would involve the therapist's intention to validate Marcus's urges, taking into consideration the concept of validation within this context (for more information on validation, refer to McMain et al., 2015, and Koerner, 2012, which discuss different levels of validation within DBT). It is important to recognize that self-harm has been Marcus's learned coping mechanism for dealing with challenging emotions. Given his history of engaging in self-harming behaviors, it is understandable that interrupting these patterns would be extremely difficult. Therefore, it is crucial to normalize and validate these urges within the context of his coping history while simultaneously motivating him to explore potential barriers that hinder alternative ways of managing these urges. On the basis of the information provided in the vignette, we are assuming that refraining from self-harm aligns with Marcus's goals.

Transference-Focused Perspective: Validate Without Reinforcing Dysfunctional Behaviors

Critically, the term *validation* may potentially be misunderstood here, at least at first glance. We assume that readers may have an initial reaction to the term validation, used in relationship with self-harming urges, in the sense of reinforcing some dysfunctional behavior. We agree, of course, that it is important not to reinforce such behaviors by offering encouragement. The term validation, specifically as used earlier—and more largely in the context of DBT—relates less to encouragement and more to self-insight. Validation, in this sense, means that one can understand the behavior, given the patient's capacities and his past habits and the short-term benefits this behavior might provide him. The patient could feel an impulse or immediate desire that explains the behavior. To validate the behavior in that light is not to congratulate him for engaging in it but to unpack why it made sense to him in the moment. Meeting the patient where he brings self-clarity to the behavior.

While this notion of validation is most associated with DBT, it is similar to how one would conceptualize an inappropriate intervention on this behavior from a TFP approach. TFP would put forth "part language," bringing both sides of the patient's experience into his awareness to help him have a more integrated and contextualized view. Essentially, part language is saying that, on the one hand, we can understand the impulse, but on the other hand, there are a whole host of negative consequences that are not aligning with the patient's overall goals or interests. Importantly, these goals or interests, although collaboratively set, are also self-set and thus not necessarily meant to be imposed on the patient by the provider. The goal of part language is to communicate that, while the impulse to engage in self-harming behavior is understandable on one level, on another level, it might be (or is) worth thinking about how to interrupt that process. As such, the use of part language "validates" the circumstances of the patient's impulses, but by reorienting him back to the collaboratively set goals, which are also his own goals, the therapist can allow him to behave in a way that is more consistent with his aspirations.

Even when we think we know what a concept means, in many cases, it is worth exploring specific meanings in different contexts. The term validation is one of those concepts. It is important to consider what we mean by using validation when describing an intervention in a particular case. It does not mean to reinforce the distortion of the thinking or the dysfunctional behavior but to convey an understanding of the problematic situation that the patient finds himself in without necessarily endorsing the solution he is using. Here, DBT would talk about "not validating the invalid" (Koerner, 2012).

Plan Analysis Perspective: Offer Strategies to Target Underlying Feelings

At this specific choice point in the narrative of Marcus's case, it may be necessary to back up a bit more. Looking back to before Marcus had these urges, we observe that when he left his two friends, he was somehow in a disconnected state and then was alone at home and engaged in different behaviors (e.g., playing piano) to reduce some of the distress. Ultimately, all this was not effective in preventing him from self-harming later in the night. What is striking in this situation is that he was completely alone and not in contact with anyone after he left his friends. This needs to be unpacked a bit more: What did he say to himself? What did he actually do? What did he feel? In this situation, it may be important for Marcus to build new skills to reach out to somebody, such as a good friend, and maybe share what he is going through, ask for help, or whatever is appropriate at that particular moment. Somehow, this would acknowledge the importance of the loneliness but also help build new competencies that he can implement before he even has the urges. These skills could prevent the urges from arising in the first place.

More generally, it is important to figure out what problem Marcus is trying to solve here. Is this a feeling of disconnection from others? Do transitions between socializing and isolation exacerbate feelings of loneliness that are present all along (or other feelings, too)? It could be that he feels disconnected from others even if he is physically with them. Marcus described this a little in the vignette when he said he spent the afternoon with his friends discussing soccer, and yet he felt somehow disconnected. It is interesting for this case to offer strategies that aim at breaking the cycle of social disconnection and self-isolation as a way to solve problems. As it happens, such a cycle is in keeping with clinical observation: Many patients with BPD report feeling disconnected from others. It would be important for this patient to learn how to go to others—friends and health care providers—and share more of his experiences with them.

"Leave Me Alone Today!" Unpacking an Interpersonally Dysregulated Situation

In the following excerpt from Session 10, Marcus describes a typical interaction with Laura in which she had suggested via text that they go to the cinema.

> So then she [Laura] texted me, and she asked me if I wanted to go to the cinema that evening. It was Saturday afternoon, and the only thing I wanted was to spend a quiet evening at home. I didn't feel like going out that evening. So somehow, I got very irritated when I saw her text, and I texted back something like, "I am sorry for today. I am tired. Leave me alone today!" I don't know why I did it that way—it does sound very harsh. So she called me, and obviously, she was upset and felt dismissed by me. I tried to explain, but somehow it didn't work. So we had this fight over the phone, which is completely ridiculous, but you know, this is what happened all the time. I am so sad about this. And I feel ashamed about being so nasty with Laura. She was right to leave me. I'm no good.

While the information provided in this choice point is meaningful and in line with what we know about Marcus, this specific example is a bit difficult because it concerns an interpersonal interaction that happened to him in real life rather than in-session with the therapist. Complicating matters further, the "yelling" in the interaction was not literal but done via text. However, this type of interaction is common, and as psychotherapists, we need to be able to analyze it.

Dialectical Behavior Perspective: Understand Precipitants Via Chain Analysis

It would be beneficial to explore the underlying factors contributing to Marcus's rejecting behavior. A useful approach in DBT is to conduct a chain analysis, as described in the scholarly writings of Linehan (1993) and Koerner (2012). Understanding the sequence of events and what led Marcus to lash out is essential in this context. The situation involving the text message provides an excellent opportunity to increase Marcus's insight and awareness of the triggers that caused his reaction to Laura's outreach. It appears that he has a history of negative treatment, which has resulted in his withdrawal from social interactions, as evidenced by his avoidance of social interactions. Therefore, it is important to reflect with Marcus on his emotional state before receiving the message. There may have been underlying emotions he was trying to protect himself from by controlling his environment, and then the text message abruptly interrupted that process. Additional details would be valuable to gain a more comprehensive understanding.

Given the limited information available about the precipitating elements of Marcus's response, we can only speculate on what might have been happening for him. One possibility is that he felt upset and ignored by his girlfriend, leading to a sense of frustration. When she reached out, his reaction might have been "too little, too late," prompting him to lash out at her. Conducting a chain analysis by asking Marcus about his emotional state before receiving the text message would provide further insight and serve as a starting point for exploration. We currently lack information about whether Marcus desired solitude, felt isolated, perceived intrusion, or simply felt angry. Understanding the sequence of events and the patient's thought process requires unpacking the information and comprehending the chain of events.

Transference-Focused Perspective: Explore Underlying Dysfunctional Thoughts and Feelings

Yet another idea on how to intervene and help understand the situation better comes from Marcus's comment, "I'm no good." There seems to be a profound feeling of treating himself with judgmental harshness, which links back to the problems related to self-criticism and low self-worth or not being good enough. Somehow, his whole sense of self was triggered by something in that interaction with his girlfriend that made him feel unworthy. That could be one explanation of what happened, and if true, we, of course, should find out what triggered it and made him react this way. The situation seems tricky for Marcus because he is trying to hold up an image of himself (and for his interaction partners) of being a lovable, correct, and good person, and this behavior contradicts that image. His other comment, "I am sorry for today," points to the idea that something preceded the text message. We may speculate that he is already harboring some active self-criticism at the moment of the message. There is an indication of dissatisfaction and criticism of his behavior over the course of the day, which should be included in the understanding of this situation.

Plan Analysis Perspective: Identify Goals and Skills for Achieving Them

One way to move forward from here, along with getting more details about the precipitating factors, is to get clarity about what Marcus really wanted in this situation. It looks like he wanted to be alone, but this might not have been as it seemed—we are not completely sure about this. If being alone was really his goal in this situation, it would be important to find out what skills would help him calmly let his girlfriend know this. Possibly, to maintain a good relationship with his girlfriend, the DBT GIVE skills (be gentle, act interested, validate, and use an easy manner) would be helpful (see Linehan, 1993, 2015, and Koerner, 2012). These skills might help him explain to her what he needs in an affirming, relationship-preserving way, not in an aggressive and rejecting way. It would take more skills to express himself in a gentle and validating way and communicate without attacking. We also need more information about the context. Were withdrawal and being alone in line with his goals? Or was he sitting alone at home because he views himself as somebody who should not be around others because he is such a "no-good" guy? Then it would be important to help him not act on the basis of these thoughts.

Yet another aspect may be an issue of control or a wish to reclaim some control. It might feel to Marcus that his relationship with his girlfriend is out of control. And, as a response, he may be asserting his need for control. He may intend to say, "No, you don't get to decide whether I am alone or whether you are in my life; I get to decide," thus telling her to go away. If this issue is relevant, it may have to be uncovered in an intervention.

Of course, these various ideas and perspectives of interventions are not necessarily mutually exclusive. Many of them could be operating at the same time and in parallel, and potentially, all interventions discussed may need to be implemented sequentially to unpack the conflictual situation with Laura and address Marcus's emotional dysregulation more generally.

SUMMARY STATEMENT: HOW TO MOVE TOWARD AN EMOTIONAL BALANCE

Emotional dysregulation is a core functional domain of personality pathology. While there is a clear consensus on this among clinical researchers and theoreticians, and it is supported by neurobiology, the treatment of dysfunctional emotional processing may take different routes. From a formulation perspective, we must answer the question of what is driving the apparent problematic emotion, the observed emotional dysregulation, or the momentary intense arousal. While the apparent emotion may have a specific quality (i.e., more or less aroused, more or less expressed) and may be described in a specific way (e.g., "I feel embarrassed"), usually there are different options for the formulation of the "driver" of this quality; the core (underlying) emotional experience may have a very different quality and may be distinct from the observed emotional experience. We agree, on the basis of Marcus's case, that the expressed emotions of embarrassment or shame may be a more secondary emotional experience, while maladaptive loneliness or core emptiness may be the driver of the emotional dysregulation. It is interesting to note that from our different formulation perspectives, we arrived at a similar conclusion regarding the focus on core emotion. This may be because most psychotherapy models treating personality pathology consider change in emotional processing to be one of the key mechanisms of change (among others; see Kramer & Timulak, 2022), which is in line with a growing body of psychotherapy research, as described earlier. Emotional processing involves asking the same questions we have asked here about which emotions are primary or secondary and which "driver" emotions underly secondary, reactive ones. While research on emotional processing is important, it tends to overlook the detailed step-by-step changes when a patient moves from emotional dysregulation to emotional balance. To understand this process at the finer grain of clinical work, we need case formulation and results from event-based process research.

The extent to which our different case formulations overlap with regard to the explanation of emotional problems may also depend on the weight attributed to different variables influencing the observed emotional problems. From a DBT perspective, there is a strong weight given to the awareness of the emotional experience (in the here and now), which helps the therapist remain focused on the quality of the emotion and how it changes from one moment to the next. From a TFP perspective, a strong weight is given to understanding the emotional experience within a dyadic interaction, where the affect may be experienced by both the subject and their interaction partner. This allows us to conceptualize additional determinants of the emotional experience, such as self-criticism, in a comprehensive way. From a plan analysis perspective, there is a strong emphasis on the instrumental components of the emotional expression, which may help us understand the link between an emotional experience or expression and an attempt to cope with a threatened self-concept or low self-worth. In conclusion, the core emotional experience driving the dysregulation needs to be unpacked and understood, and several explanatory concepts may help achieve this.

When the patient moves from emotional dysregulation to emotional balance, it may be important for the therapist to check, at each stage along the way, whether the patient is avoiding the momentary or here-and-now emotional experience, even in subtle ways. In the clinical example provided here, both the interaction via text message (where the patient "text yells" at his girlfriend) and the fact that the patient chose to describe this incident in the therapy hour may be understood as avoidance of the momentary emotional experience. Another avoidance identified in this patient along the way toward emotional balance is the presentation of "shame" as a secondary emotion. This is, of course, not an intentional avoidance but a sublimation or reexperience of the primary emotion in a different way. Therapists are encouraged to formulate these different aspects of emotional experience, recognize forms of avoidance, and move toward accessing more primary underlying emotions (i.e., loneliness in the case of Marcus).

Emotional dysregulation often takes place within an interpersonal context, making it a key double target for intervention. First, the therapist may directly intervene by helping the patient become aware of and regulate the emotional experience (e.g., from a DBT perspective, have Marcus become aware of his assumptions of being a "no-good" guy in relation to his girlfriend). Second, the therapist may intervene by helping increase awareness of the interpersonal context in which the emotional dysregulation appeared (e.g., from a TFP perspective, make Marcus aware of the interpersonal complexity of the relationship with his girlfriend and his contributions to the difficulties). Emotional dysregulation observed in the patient represents another key juncture of psychotherapeutic intervention, at which the therapist can choose between two alternative (and complementary) intervention strategies: (a) providing a structure of motivational clarification and promoting awareness of the patient's goals and needs and (b) teaching needed skills to the patient to increase their coping effectiveness in the dysregulated situation. In many clinical situations where therapists are addressing emotional dysregulation with the aim of moving toward emotional balance, they, in effect, provide both strategies. In the case of Marcus, our different intervention strategies aim at both (a) increasing Marcus's awareness and using clarification to ascertain his central goals and (b) increasing his capacity to adopt a functional behavior in a particular situation (e.g., the GIVE skills or distress tolerance techniques from DBT).

Fostering these changes takes place within a specific therapeutic relationship (see Chapter 9). It may be important to develop more research into the interplay between the therapeutic relationship and how the therapist fosters the patient's move toward emotional balance. Which aspects of the therapeutic relationship (e.g., the therapist validating the patient's experience) may help regulate the emotion? Which aspects of a responsive therapeutic relationship (e.g., the therapist focusing on the presumed underlying motive) may help increase awareness in the patient about their central goals and needs? Which aspects of relationship interpretations (e.g., the therapist noting the current interaction as a repetition of past affective experiences and interactions) may help increase awareness and regulation? It may also be important to differentiate "good process" indicators from "less good" process indicators. The notion of validation may provide an example: Which aspects of therapist "validation" inadvertently reinforce the patient's distorted view of their experience? More focused research in a variety of therapeutic approaches in observing the in-session behaviors of patients with personality pathology and their therapists may help gain insight into these open questions on how to foster emotional balance in these treatments.

5 MOVING FROM PROBLEMATIC SOCIAL INTERACTIONS TO INTERPERSONAL EFFECTIVENESS

Patients with personality disorders often present with interpersonal difficulties and disturbed social functioning; they frequently seek treatment with complaints about problems in their relationships, including a lack of close friendships. This chapter explores the mechanisms of change related to disturbed interpersonal difficulties (e.g., interpersonal concerns, dependency, fear of rejection) and social functioning (e.g., number of friends) and examines how therapists can focus on these dimensions to foster the capacity for interpersonal relatedness and social competencies. We begin by summarizing the empirical evidence related to mechanisms of change relevant to interpersonal relatedness and social functioning. Next, we present the case of Janet, a woman whose treatment primarily focused on her difficulties in interpersonal relatedness and improving her social functioning.[1] Our case discussion focuses on how to foster trust in relationships, including the therapeutic relationship; address a person's sense of "not belonging in the world"; and alter the underlying problematic perception of being alone.

---

[1]The case of Janet has been modified to disguise the patient's identity and protect her confidentiality.

https://doi.org/10.1037/0000388-006
Understanding Mechanisms of Change in Psychotherapies for Personality Disorders, by U. Kramer, K. N. Levy, and S. McMain

We discuss how to bring about therapeutic change in deficits in social functioning to increase interpersonal effectiveness and improve social functioning. The chapter concludes with a summary of our understanding of how to foster change in interpersonal and social dimensions by integrating knowledge derived from research, theory, and our clinical perspectives as they are applied to an individual case.

EMPIRICAL SUPPORT FOR MECHANISMS OF CHANGE: DISTURBED INTERPERSONAL RELATEDNESS AND SOCIAL FUNCTIONING

Broadly defined, *social cognitive processing* refers to the ability to process social information and, therefore, it is vital to how people read and respond to the emotions and intentions of others (Henry et al., 2015). It has received recent attention in the clinical and empirical literature. Social cognitive processing has been operationalized using a number of different concepts, including theory of mind, mentalizing (including reflective functioning), and metacognition. Social cognitive processing underlies interpersonal relatedness, social functioning, and self-concept and is known to be involved in deficits seen in individuals with personality disorders; hence, it has implications for therapeutic intervention.

Several studies have examined whether constructs related to social cognitive processing are mechanisms of change in therapy for personality disorders. Several studies have examined changes in mentalizing and reflective functioning, which are operationalized as the capacity to understand and reflect on one's own and others' mental states. Specifically, two controlled studies investigated the effectiveness of transference-focused psychotherapy (TFP) for borderline personality disorder (BPD). Levy et al. (2006) showed that TFP was associated with large increases in the quality of reflective functioning, as observed in independent adult attachment interviews, and with changes in attachment status. In a study of 104 patients with BPD receiving either TFP or treatment by experienced therapists, Fischer-Kern et al. (2015) found that the TFP group was associated with improvements in reflective functioning and that these improvements, in turn, predicted improvements in personality organization.

In a study of 175 patients with BPD receiving long-term psychodynamic therapy that examined whether changes in mentalization are associated with treatment outcome, De Meulemeester et al. (2018) found that improvements in mentalizing capacities, defined as increased certainty about the mental states of others, predicted the rate of improvement on symptom distress. A study of reflective functioning by Chiesa et al. (2021) examined 111 patients with a personality disorder who received either one of two specialist psychotherapy programs (long-term residential or a step-down model) or a generalist approach over a 2-year period. The step-down specialist program was found to be more effective in improving reflective functioning than the other treatments, and these changes, in turn, predicted improvements in social and global functioning outcomes. In another study of psychodynamic therapy for BPD with comorbid substance dependence, Möller et al. (2017) found that the therapeutic focus on actively fostering mentalizing was related to patients' in-session quality of mentalizing.

Difficulties in interpersonal relatedness may also be operationalized using the pervasiveness of interpersonal patterns, such as in research on the core conflictual relationship theme. In a study of individuals with BPD undergoing good psychiatric management treatment, Kramer, Beuchat, et al. (2022) observed that changes in the pervasiveness of representations of conflictual themes are related to a person's reaction to interpersonal dynamics. These changes in representations of core conflicts were also related to decreased borderline symptoms at the end of therapy. Interestingly, a study of long-term psychotherapy in a large heterogeneous sample of individuals with personality disorders ($N = 382$) found that changes in patients' interpersonal patterns were related to reductions in symptom severity (Babl et al., 2022). The relation between such changes in interpersonal patterns and outcome was explained by therapist interventions that addressed interpersonal patterns as they occurred in session between the therapist and patient.

Change in metacognition, a construct related to mentalization and reflective functioning, has also been investigated. In a study using observer-rated methodology applied to early and late sessions, Maillard et al. (2019) found that the ability to differentiate between representations and reality increased over the course of treatment and that these improvements predicted symptom decreases at 6-month follow-up.

While it can be argued that changes in internal representations related to social interactions may be targeted mostly in psychodynamic and humanistic treatments, it remains an open question whether these changes may also be observed in behavior therapy, such as dialectical behavior therapy (DBT). Bedics et al. (2012) addressed this question by focusing on the quality of introject (using the Structural Analysis of Social Behavior methodology) and its changes over the course of DBT and found that patients reported increased self-affirmation, self-love, and self-protection, and decreased self-attack after behavior treatment, which was not found in the comparator condition. Specific aspects of views of the therapist (seeing them as more affirming and protecting) predicted a decrease in self-harm behavior at the end of therapy.

Other related research has explored changes to cognitive structures, biases, and heuristics in psychotherapy for people with personality disorders (e.g., Arntz et al., 2012; Keller et al., 2018; Kramer & Golam, 2019). Finally, change in theory of mind has been explored with neurobehavioral data. A few studies have shown that the effects of therapy are associated with changes in the orbitofrontal and anterior cingulate cortices and the ventral striatum, the areas of the brain related to theory of mind and complex task processing (Kramer, Kolly, et al., 2018; O'Neill et al., 2015).

In summary, the empirical literature provides preliminary evidence confirming that changes in constructs related to social cognitive processing, such as reflective functioning, mentalization, theory of mind, interpersonal patterns, and metacognition, are associated with treatment effects in psychotherapy for personality disorders.

THE CASE OF JANET

Janet is a 40-year-old single woman who lives alone and has never been in a romantic relationship. She is employed full-time as an accountant at a large firm in a metropolitan city and works long hours (55+ per week), which she said helps to distract her from her chronic feelings of loneliness. Janet reported feeling chronically depressed and "miserable." Over the past several years, she often felt sad due to feeling alone. To "turn off" ruminative depressive thoughts about being alone, she drinks wine or engages in work to numb her feelings and distract her mind. She currently drinks two glasses of wine on weeknights and five to six glasses per evening on weekends.

With respect to her personal history, Janet had a lonely childhood in a cold and unhappy family environment. She reported that both parents were emotionally unsupportive, and she has no memories of ever being emotionally comforted by them. Her parents frequently quarreled or isolated themselves from each other and their children, and she could not recount any positive memories of time spent as a family. She denied any history of physical or sexual abuse. She recalled spending much of her childhood entertaining herself alone in her room. She had few friends and reported that by age 8, she had started having thoughts of suicide. Her workaholic father was often not present, and his absence, coupled with her mother's lack of attention, left her feeling flawed and undesirable. She was 10 when her parents divorced, at which time she and her older sister moved into a new home with their mother, and she ended contact with her father. Although she had never been fond of him, she felt a tremendous sense of aloneness on his departure and stated, "My world shattered when he left." She portrayed her mother as an emotionally fragile self-absorbed woman who would often isolate herself in her room when in a depressed mood. Her sister, who was 6 years older, escaped by becoming involved in social activities outside the home. Janet was always jealous of her sister, who she felt was favored over herself, and wished that she too could have escaped the emotionally oppressive home environment.

Janet has difficult relationships with her family. She is in frequent contact with her mother and sister, but these interactions are often tense and conflictual. She reported that her family says she has an explosive temper, and they often accuse her of being selfish. She fights with her sister and brother-in-law frequently; arguments are usually triggered by her perception that others do not value her or support her enough. She talks on the phone with her mother regularly but says she feels unsupported and hurt by her mother, who usually sides with Janet's sister. Janet's anger outbursts have contributed to strains in her family relationships; she has gone for months without speaking to her family.

With respect to social relationships, Janet has no close friends. She has maintained occasional contact with some childhood friends but does not feel close to any of them. She works long hours and stated that due to her work demands, she has little time to connect with people socially. In social encounters, she usually perceives herself as not fitting in, as being excluded, and ignored. Her perceptions of others contribute to feelings of anger toward people. At her workplace, she avoids personal conversations and engages with colleagues only on work-related matters. Although she is perceived as hard working and productive, she has not been promoted and has received feedback from her manager that her communication style is too abrupt and abrasive.

Janet has a strong sense of being alone in the world, and although she is successful at work, she feels an overall sense of misery in her life. Diagnostically, she meets the criteria for BPD, alcohol abuse, and dysthymia. From a personality trait dimensional perspective, she presents as high on negative emotionality with a predominant depressive mood and high on introversion characterized by an avoidant style in social interactions.

Janet is highly dependent on her therapy for social connection, looking forward to her sessions every week and becoming anxious and irritable if the therapist takes a vacation or broaches the topic of treatment termination. She told her therapist, "You're the only person in my world that I talk to." Before her current therapist, she had been seeing a cognitive behavior therapist for 15 years, but he recently retired, and Janet still harbors tremendous anger toward him for his perceived abandonment. She emphasized that no treatment has helped her, and she has little confidence that it will now. At the same time, she conveyed that it was important to her to have a therapist who would be available to her and commit to working with her for an extended period. She was highly reluctant to discuss the length of therapy.

In her initial sessions, Janet presented in a businesslike manner and appeared guarded and mistrustful. She rarely smiled, and her facial expression seemed predisposed to be a natural scowl. She has a passive-aggressive manner that makes it appear she is angry at people and dislikes them. Janet generally expressed hostility and disapproval toward the therapist throughout the therapeutic process, including in a later session in which she complained that the therapist did not have a white noise machine and all other therapists have one (this incident is reviewed in more detail later as a key clinical choice point).

CASE FORMULATION: IDENTIFYING DETERMINANTS OF PROBLEMATIC INTERPERSONAL BEHAVIORS

Our case formulations aim to understand the determinants of this patient's problematic interpersonal and social behaviors. Next, we outline our three perspectives on the case of Janet, followed by a general synthesis of our ideas.

Plan Analysis Formulation: Motive-Oriented Relationship

In Janet's case, interpersonal and social problems are at the forefront. Janet appears to have intense feelings of loneliness in reaction to several social cues. Janet mentioned that she has no friends or anyone to whom she feels close. Given the case description, we speculate that Janet struggles to have solid psychological ground to stand on. In various instances, she feels rejected, excluded, or dismissed in social interactions. To compensate for some of these deeper vulnerabilities, Janet appears to exhibit a variety of coping strategies— some strategies, such as an overly professional and business style of presentation, may have advantages.

From a plan analysis approach, one question concerns the purpose of Janet's business-style self-presentation. How does it relate to her loneliness and fear of losing a significant relationship, including the one with the therapist? What is the purpose of this presentation of the self? Janet appears to be performing— or sometimes overperforming—in her job, which may allow her to avoid being confronted by feeling loneliness or exclusion from others. It may be a coping strategy that corresponds to a plan, such as needing to be "a strong worker." This presentation may serve the purpose or goal of avoiding feelings of loneliness or avoiding admitting being vulnerable. She copes with stress by drinking alcohol, possibly to avoid feeling lonely and confronting her somewhat "unconstructed" self and the fundamental threat of being alone.

Notably, Janet avoided discussions about treatment termination, which were difficult to pursue with her. Janet quickly launched into complaints about her interpersonal relationships and subtly attacked her therapist. Her hostility may be a way of coping with her inability to connect with herself and use her inner experiences, wishes, desires, and feelings to feel accomplished.

Janet also appeared to express hostility in the therapeutic relationship (e.g., complaining that the therapist does not have a white noise machine) and her relationship with close others (e.g., anger outbursts and not speaking with her sister and mother). In the therapy context, Janet presented as somebody who seemed to be well-versed in therapy and the protection of privacy (i.e., by using white noise machines). What is the purpose of Janet stating, "Other therapists use white noise machines"? It may be that she aimed to highlight that this therapist does not do what everybody else seems to do to protect a patient's privacy. One could hypothesize that Janet's insistence on these aspects may be understood in the context of a plan such as "present as somebody who is knowledgeable about therapy" or "check whether this therapist is aware of some potential flaws." A possible interpersonal message from the client to the therapist could be, "I have done cognitive behavior therapy [CBT; or another therapy] before," which could be interpreted as a subtle implication of expertise or knowledge in the field. As such, we can speculate that these interactions allow Janet to present as an expert in certain areas and to highlight her expertise. This behavior may serve Janet's supposedly central purpose of attempting to receive particularly effective treatment. An additional motive behind these behaviors and plans may be the regulation of closeness (i.e., her expression of neediness) and interpersonal distance.

The question at this juncture becomes which motive is acceptable in this situation. From a motive-oriented therapeutic relationship perspective, the therapist may deliberately focus on (or reinforce) the underlying acceptable motives in a plan structure while avoiding the risk of reinforcing problematic plans, behaviors, and experiences. For the therapist to use the motive-oriented therapeutic relationship implies that certain aspects can be attended to in a complementary fashion; the unproblematic aspects high in the hierarchy of plans—the therapist should not attend directly to other aspects of the patient presentation—and the problematic aspects low in the hierarchy of plans and behaviors.

Emphasizing the absence of the noise machine and the fact that she had therapy before may contribute to Janet's global presentation as someone who is knowledgeable about ethical boundaries of psychotherapy (i.e., possibly to a similar extent as the therapist) and how therapy works. This may be a way for her to present herself as an expert on an interpersonal level. An interpersonal focus may not be helpful because it will not allow her to focus on her sense of self and examine her doubts and lack of clarity and inconsistencies about herself. The overall goal of Janet's plans and behaviors may be to enhance a sense of control or ensure that she receives a particularly effective treatment. The question remains how inferences about Janet's underlying plan can inform the therapist's interventions.

Focusing on the underlying motive(s) may be a way of making use of the contents of the plan analysis. For example, a therapist who responds by saying, "You know, CBT does not always work," or "Noise machines are not necessarily effective," may be frustrating to Janet and miss the mark. In addition, such responses may activate her negative expectations about interpersonal interactions. She may feel rejected and more alone, which may lie at the core of her problems in functioning. Janet may regard a therapist who is not warm enough as rejecting, unlike a therapist who responds by saying, "You know, it is so important that you pointed out the noise machine to me [or about having had CBT before]. If you agree, I will try to provide my best understanding of you and help you move forward in your life [or help you receive the best possible treatment]." Being complementary to her motive—perhaps the desire for a helpful treatment—is the guiding principle in working with this patient.

Transference-Focused Formulation: Rigid Self-Representation

From a TFP case formulation, Janet has a rather rigid representation of others vis-à-vis herself and possibly a rigid representation of herself as well. A goal of therapy would entail helping her develop more nuanced, flexible, and richer representations of herself and others that would allow her to consider more possibilities, have more access to the richer and more nuanced representations, and as a result, develop a better capacity to tolerate ambiguity in relationships. From a TFP perspective, we would hypothesize that the latter is one of the main issues: She has so much intolerance of ambiguity that she needs to rigidly hold onto these ideas about who she is, who other people are, and how they treat her. This may be her way of gaining some control over situations in which she otherwise feels so out of control. Although we typically would not comment about early childhood in the therapy, we might hypothesize that, as a child, Janet did not have any control over engaging her parents and sister in a way that brought connection and comfort. Such experiences may have been regularly repeated over the years. Now, as then, Janet might have learned to erect rigid views of "how things are" and to try to control people in an effort to provide some stability. But of course, she cannot control them, so there is some vacillation between feeling out of control and trying to put people into boxes that would give her a sense of security and control. These two representations of herself and others are inconsistent and lead her to feel and act in wildly different ways, neither of which are effective.

From an attachment theory perspective, Janet may vacillate between the classically insecure-preoccupied and dismissing patterns or states of mind. Preoccupied states of mind are characterized by desiring closeness with others and emotional activation. People with this attachment state of mind can be needy but not necessarily compliant with the frame of treatment and therapy goals. They want to be close to others but may have a strong desire to control what that closeness looks like. In contrast, those with dismissing attachment or in a dismissing state of mind with respect to attachment are often resistant to starting treatment and have difficulty asking for help and may retreat from help when offered (Levy & Kelly, 2009). Whereas those with preoccupied attachment patterns may leave therapists feeling overwhelmed, those with dismissive attachment may leave therapists feeling rejected and excluded from the patient's life.

Although most individuals present with an organized pattern of attachment (e.g., secure, preoccupied, dismissing), we have found that many patients with personality disorders vacillate between these two states of mind, psychologically approaching the therapist, often in an engulfing way, and then psychologically withdrawing from the therapist. The admixture of these attachment states often results in an angry or hostile withdrawal from others, including the therapist. When these individuals want others to act in certain ways for them and that does not happen, they swing to the avoidance pole, not in a purely unemotional detached way but with a lot of hostility. In addition, at least from her description, Janet's parents seem to have met this profile as well, however, this is unclear because some patients describe their parents in particular ways that may not correspond to reality. Sometimes, when a therapist meets a patient's parents, they do not conform to expectations based on the patient's description. This is why focusing on the here and now of the interaction between the therapist and patient is viewed as the most fruitful material for the therapy. To the degree that the therapist is integrated and thus knows how they behaved in session, any distortions, even subtle and mild ones, can be examined, understood, and resolved. These representations, however developed, although most likely from real experience, are then

rigidly held and applied (or projected) onto others in subsequent interactions. When such schemas are activated in session, they are ripe for reflection
because they have an in vivo relevance.

Dialectical Behavior Formulation: Internalized Emotional Invalidation

In the context of DBT, psychopathology is viewed as deficits in emotion regulation capacities, which contribute to the avoidance and escape from productive emotional experiences. With this perspective in mind, our formulation of
Janet's case begins by exploring how deficits in emotion regulation underlie
the development and maintenance of her presenting problems. Maladaptive
behaviors and dysfunctional self-perceptions often arise when individuals
exhibit a tendency to avoid and escape primary automatic emotional experiences. These deficits in emotion regulation capacities emerge through the
dynamic interplay of biological and psychosocial factors.

According to my assessment, Janet experienced significant emotional invalidation from her parents during childhood, which likely contributed to the
aforementioned problematic processes. Her mother's mental health issues,
characterized by frequent withdrawal, isolation, and depression, suggest a
potential heritable component to Janet's emotionally vulnerable constitution.
In terms of environmental factors, Janet's parents spent little time with her,
leading to her feelings of isolation and a perceived lack of interest and affec-
tion. Janet perceived her parents' behavior as highly emotionally invalidating,
which had detrimental consequences for her, including overwhelming, painful
emotions. The absence of nurturance and emotional support prevented her
from learning effective ways to soothe herself and tolerate distressing emotions. In addition, the lack of validation and empathy from others hindered her
ability to acknowledge and validate her own emotional experiences, cutting
her off from important adaptive information.

At the core of Janet's presenting problems is her profound sense of loneliness, which contributes to feelings of fear and sadness. This intense and
painful sense of aloneness, extending beyond the physical aspect, is common
among individuals diagnosed with BPD, particularly those who have experienced significant traumatic invalidation. Janet's feelings of misery associated
with spending time alone without support can be traced back to her early
childhood experiences, likely creating a sense of terror for a young child.

Janet exhibits a range of severe problems, including depressed mood,
alcohol abuse, anger outbursts, chronic suicidal thoughts, limited social connections, and excessive work engagement. Many of these behaviors serve
as escape or avoidance mechanisms to evade underlying fear, sadness, and

shame. For instance, Janet engages in interpersonal avoidance by avoiding meaningful connections with coworkers, refraining from small talk, and keeping conversations focused solely on work. While these avoidance behaviors temporarily shield her from adverse emotions, they exacerbate her problems by intensifying her feelings of aloneness, isolation, and sadness.

Furthermore, Janet's highly judgmental self-concept perpetuates her problems. She holds negative beliefs about herself, such as, "There's something wrong with me," "I'm not acceptable to others," and "I don't belong." She expects others to reject her and firmly believes they are not interested in being around her. This chronically negative self-narrative stems from her emotionally invalidating experiences. Janet's self-criticism and negative narrative likely developed as a coping mechanism in response to emotional trauma. By blaming herself and viewing herself as flawed, she gained a sense of control over an otherwise uncontrollable situation, helping her escape overwhelming aversive emotions such as shame and sadness. Self-blame provides a temporary sense of control, especially when she internalizes thoughts such as "It was my fault," "What did I do wrong?" "If only I were a better kid," and "If only I were more likable, my parents would pay attention to me." However, these judgmental thoughts perpetuate her problems in the long run. For instance, when she believes others dislike her and do not want to be around her, she withdraws socially to protect herself from anticipated rejection and abandonment. Her judgments of herself and others also contribute to her isolation from others.

Janet's struggles involve both internal and external triggers that activate her profound sense of aloneness. Criticism from others or reminders of loss tend to evoke underlying painful emotions and intensify her feelings of isolation. In response to these aversive emotions, Janet engages in behaviors that serve as a means of escape or avoidance. Weekends are particularly challenging for her because she perceives others as being occupied with friends and family, further amplifying her sense of aloneness. To manage these emotions, she resorts to alcohol consumption and excessive work.

It is crucial to prioritize the elimination of problematic behaviors in Janet's treatment plan. Addressing behaviors such as drinking, excessive work, avoidance of social interactions, and self-criticism is of utmost importance because they serve as avenues for escaping her underlying aversive emotions. The initial step in Janet's journey toward transformation involves fostering an environment that allows and tolerates these emotions. By creating space for Janet to acknowledge and experience emotions such as loss, disappointment, and powerlessness without resorting to escape or avoidance, she can begin the process of transforming them in a healthier and more adaptive manner.

Toward a Common Formulation

Despite the diversity of our theoretical approaches, our formulations have some common ideas. One similarity in our perspectives is the idea that a major part of Janet's presenting issues can be traced back to a range of invalidating childhood experiences. For example, we agreed that Janet's absence of connection to her parents and lack of a sense of security and safety in the family environment contributed to her poor self-construct.

Another shared understanding in our perspectives is the centrality of the idea that Janet's psychopathological behaviors (e.g., anger, drinking, a rigid interpersonal style of engagement) are self-protective mechanisms that developed as a means to protect her from experiencing more vulnerable emotions and experiences. However, while these problematic behaviors are conceptualized from the lens of adaptive coping, it is also understood that they are currently perpetuating her difficulties and failures in the interpersonal and social domains of functioning.

In terms of our conceptualizations, all methods go beyond the diagnosis and presenting problems in an effort to understand the mechanisms that have produced Janet's presenting problems. The TFP and plan analytic methods both emphasize that Janet's interpersonal problems and social deficits result directly from a rigid and poorly defined sense of self. TFP additionally emphasizes her rigid and inflexible self-representations, while the plan analytic method incorporates the notion that these problems result directly from a deficient self-concept. The DBT method differs from the others by emphasizing that Janet's negative narrative, which forms the basis of her self-construct, is secondary to an emotional problem and is functioning to help her avoid activating underlying painful emotional experiences.

The plan analytic and DBT approaches emphasize the centrality of emotion in the formulation. Both stress the importance of avoided emotional needs and the therapeutic value of helping the patient not interrupt and avoid primary adaptive emotional experiences. They conceptualize Janet's primary emotional problem as a fear of loneliness and share the notion that her interpersonal style, impulsive behaviors, and general ways of coping are operating as a means to manage her underlying core fear of aloneness. For example, Janet's rigid, businesslike, expertlike stance is viewed as a way of bolstering her sense of control, avoiding intimacy, and managing her underlying vulnerable experience of loneliness.

In terms of the implications of our formulations for intervention, we agree that Janet's interpersonal and social problems should be a central focus of intervention. To tackle these problems, the plan analytic and DBT approaches share the view that her underlying feelings of loneliness need to be a focus in the intervention. There is also agreement across our perspectives that Janet's problems are multilayered and the interventions will need to address all the layers of emotional needs.

While our diverse formulations have similarities in both perspectives and implications for intervention, there are other notable areas of difference. An adapted DBT approach may focus on processing problematic emotions stemming from Janet's experiences of traumatic invalidation. The TFP formulation may focus more on Janet's imprecise or biased representations of self-in-interaction-with-others leading to her difficulty in interpersonal interactions. A plan analytic formulation may conceptualize Janet's coping behaviors as plans serving overarching motives (e.g., a motive to avoid feeling her vulnerable sense of self or a motive to request a particularly effective treatment), which the therapist should attend to in a complementary fashion.

CHOICE POINTS AND OPPORTUNITIES FOR CHANGE

In the next section, the treatment implications of our case formulations are discussed within the context of therapists' decision-making process on how to respond to specific moments in therapy. We identified three choice points that required the therapist to respond based on their case formulation and the context of a specific moment in therapy. Three choice points are discussed: (a) Janet described her ingrained perception that others reject her, (b) Janet stated that she is all alone and does not belong, and (c) Janet mildly complained about the therapist not having a white noise machine. We conclude by summarizing the decision making that guides our selection for specific interventions in response to a given moment in therapy. Table 5.1 synthesizes generic and approach-specific strategies that therapists might use, as well as relevant patient processes, in the three choice points presented in this chapter.

"I Have No Friends!": Addressing Perceptions That Others Are Rejecting

Janet presented to session in a typical manner. She expressed feelings of bitterness toward others whom she perceived as having been unsupportive. In the current situation, she had taken recent steps to expand her social network and was rejected by someone she was trying to befriend. She appeared depressed, hopeless, and helpless. In a complaining and bitter tone, she stated,

> It's been a bad week. It's the same old, same old all the time. The only friend that I had no longer wants anything to do with me, and now I have nobody. I push myself to have these relationships. All I got back from this supposed

TABLE 5.1. How to Foster a Path to Interpersonal Effectiveness

Generic therapist interventions	Specific therapist interventions	Patient processes
Choice point: Addressing perceived rejection		
• Convey understanding and clarify perception.	• Focus on the underlying motive.	• Become aware of their needs.
• Manage alliance ruptures.	• Confront patient behavior.	• Become aware of their choices.
• Foster reality testing.	• Check the facts.	• Learn to describe (vs. judge).
• Promote awareness.	• Foster awareness of perceptions.	
• Challenge distorted perceptions.	• Change patient perceptions.	• Become aware of perceptions.
• Clarify the goal or mission.	• Increase the motivation to change.	• Restructure perceptions.
		• Remain committed to change.
Choice point: Addressing the sense of not belonging		
• Offer acceptance.	• Validate experience.	• Feel "normalized."
• Change the emotion.	• Increase exposure to avoided emotion.	• Feel and change emotion.
• Transform the emotion.		
• Provide a corrective experience.	• Foster new emotional experiences.	• Feel new emotion in session.
• Provide clarification.	• Affirm their presence in the room.	• Feel connected.
	• Offer process guidance.	
Choice point: Addressing in-session complaints		
• Foster corrective experience.	• Focus on the underlying motive.	• Have new experiences.
• Contain emotion.	• Foster trust in the therapy relationship.	• Develop reflectivity.
	• Focus on the task at hand.	• Refocus attention.

friend is, "I don't care," and "I have no compassion for you." She hasn't been a very good friend to me. It's been like trying to squeeze love from a stone with her. She doesn't seem to understand that I'm unhealthy and need support.

How does a therapist decide how to intervene at this moment in therapy in view of the evidence that this woman has an ingrained view that other people reject her and judge her and that she is helpless to avoid the rejection of others?

Plan Analysis Perspective: Motive-Oriented Therapeutic Relationship

As a first step, when Janet says something like, "I have nobody; I pushed myself in these relationships!" it is important to make sense of this statement in terms of the case formulation. It may be that relationships seem unstable to this person because of her traumatic history of being left alone so often and a sense of insecurity, including in the relationship with the therapist, which is also something that will end at one point. Janet may be afraid that the therapist may reject her at one point.

An intervention consistent with a plan analytic approach and motive-oriented therapeutic relationship, as discussed previously (but extending its principles a bit), is to say, "It seems like it's so important that you prevent people from leaving you or people leaving you at one point, including me, the therapist. This could interfere with what is happening between you and me, so I want to make sure you feel welcome in this relationship." The therapist may put that statement on the table as an intervention; it could become a central social interaction problem and how the patient and therapist together as a team may be addressing it. By doing this in a proactive way, before a relationship rupture occurs, the therapist may model collaboration—or "coax" the interaction partner into some kind of collaboration—by focusing on the behavior underlying the motive. From a different psychotherapy framework, the Cognitive Behavioral Analysis System for Psychotherapy (McCullough et al., 2014), the aforementioned elaboration is consistent with the proactive evocation of the transference hypothesis in the treatment of patients with chronic depression.

The underlying content of Janet saying "I have no friends" may, in this case, be her chronic sense of loneliness, echoing a chilly feeling when we imagine this lonely small girl without anybody in her family responding to her—this steel-cold and neglectful context. Her presentation of herself makes sense in this context and is a way to cope with this loneliness (e.g., Janet's sometimes bossy or business-type way of interaction). In many situations, Janet may feel or anticipate that people are rejecting her and so does some preemptive action that prevents it from happening. Without these preemptive actions, the situation may bring back all the painful, traumatic memories of what she had gone through.* She has been developing all these assumptions—that relationships may be unstable (as affective schema) or even that relationships are there to hurt her, reject her, or criticize her in some ways. Alternatively, her bossy style may serve to maintain her control over the interaction to prevent her from feeling like a victim in the interaction. These contents need to be clarified as soon as the patient shows readiness to do so.

From a motive-oriented therapeutic relationship perspective, it seems crucial to understand her statement, "I have no friends!" as a potential problem for the therapeutic relationship, but it may also be risky to intervene directly with such a focus on the current therapeutic relationship. The therapist may state, "I see your pain of not having real friends around you. One thing I understand from what you are saying is that to have trustworthy relationships is super important to you. If you agree, let's work together to understand better how you can trust people more." Understanding that she has these difficult interactions and marking them as such is important. As a result, Janet may feel rejected or act in a businesslike or bossy way or even a bit aggressively. This may be a key area of any relationship Janet is in and provides a sense of safety to address the underlying motives—what Janet craved in her upbringing and never received. Addressing these motives and giving and repairing some of what she never received in her relationships may prevent a later misunderstanding or potential ruptures in the therapeutic relationship and fundamentally support healing the trauma by fostering corrective relationship experiences.

Transference-Focused Perspective: Explore the Patient's Perception of the Therapeutic Relationship

A TFP perspective shares ideas similar to a plan analytic method, however, there are some important differences. It is unclear whether this topic should be brought into the therapeutic relationship so early, but it would have to be part of the discussion. Janet described consistent narrative themes of people frequently leaving her in the "same old, same old" way and not being able to count on people. However, the therapeutic relationship is different from other relationships because therapy is time limited in terms of the length of sessions and the length of a course of therapy. Janet may also be asking herself questions such as, "What's the use? Why am I investing in this if this is gonna be ripped from me, just like everything else?"

To address this issue, it would be important to have some concrete manifestations of the problem, such as references and utterances that may be consistent with the topic. Exploration may also be used when something is interfering with the process, such as when Janet talks about trivial things, and the therapist thinks the reason is that Janet is concerned about the therapeutic relationship and what it means to be engaged in the therapy. Another question involves whether Janet is picking the wrong people, actively pushing people away, or whether it was just bad luck. This process needs to be explored and clarified. It is important to see whether the material Janet brought up fits with other material from the session.

When Janet says, "It's the same old, same old. . . . I have nobody. I push myself to have these relationships," that forming a satisfying intimate relationship is "like trying to squeeze love from a stone," and that her friend "doesn't seem to understand that I'm unhealthy and need support," it may indicate that she wishes she had someone to take care of her in the way a sick patient might want a nurse or a child might want a parent. This may not be what the therapist should say, but the theme should be explored. The therapist may want to say, "It sounds like you're aware of your desire for closeness and intimacy and feel as if others don't understand that or really care about that aspect of you. Do I understand that correctly?"

What Janet expressed may also be understood in the context of the transference relationship. The therapist may say, "You know, what you're describing with your friend seems to me to be a kind of dynamic you've experienced before with other people. It is the idea of once bitten, twice shy. You push yourself to do these things, and then you get bitten again. And I'm wondering if you're looking for support and people don't see it. I'm wondering if it's not exactly the same thing but something like it that's worth our thinking about together."

Dialectical Behavior Perspective: Help Patients Observe Thoughts and Perceptions

The therapist can begin by acknowledging Janet's perception of being rejected by others and her recurring feelings of hopelessness within relationships. Janet's belief that she does not belong and her view of others as rejecting her is a reflection of her deep-seated experiences. It is understandable that she feels alone and saddened by these perceptions. In response to Janet's comment, a DBT therapist would adopt a compassionate stance and respond by validating what is reasonable or what makes sense about the patient's perceptions, considering her childhood experiences. The therapist would recognize that Janet's present reality parallels her past emotional experiences.

During the session, the therapist should guide Janet in mindfully observing her thoughts and perceptions to increase self-awareness. Given the deeply ingrained nature of Janet's perceptions, caution should be exercised when challenging her cognitions. Traditional cognitive restructuring techniques may be experienced as invalidating and could activate the same patterns of perception and relationship dynamics within the therapeutic relationship (e.g., "My therapist is rejecting me"). Instead, the therapist can employ lighter forms of cognitive restructuring by helping Janet pay attention to her thoughts and their impact on her emotions and behavior. Validating statements and simple reflections can support this process.

It is also important for the therapist to assist Janet in distinguishing between the facts of a situation and her assumptions. When Janet expresses feeling rejected, the therapist can encourage her to describe what actually happened and how she responded. People often hold assumptions about others' motives, and thoughts can be intertwined with inferences that go beyond factual evidence. The therapist can gently highlight these assumptions, taking into account Janet's sensitivity to perceived rejection. Strong challenges to her perceptions are likely to be perceived as threatening. As long as the patient feels safe, the therapist can explore Janet's perceptions and help her recognize their presence in broader patterns. By highlighting the similarity of her thoughts across various situations, the therapist can support Janet in gaining distance from her thoughts and perceptions, helping her realize they are part of a recurring problematic narrative that becomes activated in relationships. Janet's negative narrative likely stems from her emotionally invalidating environment. Introducing a skill from Bohus's DBT-PTSD manual (Bohus et al., 2019), such as "change your glasses," could be useful in helping Janet recognize when past emotional experiences are being reactivated in the present and learn to differentiate between the two.

The therapist may invite Janet to replay her interaction with her "friend" in a detailed chain analysis, aiming to increase her insight and awareness of her responses. Through this process, Janet can become more attuned to her micro-expressions and subtle communicative behaviors in her interactions with others. The more Janet subscribes to the belief that she is being rejected, the more likely her negative thoughts will influence her behavior and interactions, leading to withdrawal or increased hostility. Janet may exhibit subtle nonverbal cues and hostility toward others without being fully aware of it. For instance, a scowl on her face may cause others to withdraw or respond in an unfriendly manner. It is also important to assess how Janet's interpersonal behavior contributes to others' withdrawal behaviors, especially if she enters relationships with a high need for support.

Another Transference-Focused Perspective: Distinguishing Reality From Perceptions

Clarifying the details of what actually happened is important because while it is likely that Janet has experienced repeated rejections, it is also quite possible that Janet has seen rejection in experiences that might not be objectively a rejection. It would be important to clarify and, possibly, gently and respectfully challenge such perceptions. In this situation, when the therapist aims at even slightly challenging or uncovering some of these issues, it may happen, of course, that the patient does not follow the therapist's thoughts. Nevertheless, this disagreement may lead to important conversations. The fact is that Janet may rigidly reject the therapist's ideas, and she may even express that she does not like the therapist.

Another way of approaching this dilemma, from a TFP perspective, is to adopt a nonjudgmental stance and see if the therapist and patient can understand what is going on so Janet can choose how she wants to proceed. She may choose to continue with rigid rejection, or another option might be available. If the patient is reluctant, the therapist may say, "It's interesting that you perceive my wanting to stop and think about this as if I were attacking you and blaming you. If someone were observing us, they might think that it is you who is attacking me by the way you said it. I think it's worth our thinking about again—not judging but understanding because, you know, this may be the kind of dynamic that's happening with friends that pushes people away at times." Here it might be important to be concrete and explain examples the patient has shared that are consistent with this.

A Clarification-Oriented Perspective: Content, Process, and Relationship

From a clarification-oriented perspective (incorporating the motive-oriented therapeutic relationship described earlier; Sachse, 2020), it sounds like other challenges may emerge in the therapeutic interaction—one related to unshared focus (i.e., a problem in process) and one related to not liking the therapist (i.e., a problem in a relationship). Here we may refer to Sachse's (2020) three levels of understanding a patient's problem: content, process, and relationship. This distinction is relevant because the theory predicts that problems on the levels of process and relationship take precedence over declared content. When working on the level of the content, the challenge is often with patients like Janet, whose beliefs and perceptions of the world, based on problematic processes or relationships, are so ingrained and firmly held that any suggestion of an alternative way of looking at things is often quickly rejected. Everything is quickly seen and judged through that lens. If the therapist does not agree with the patient, the therapist becomes part of the distorted perception. Work on this content may become a relationship crisis because patients may feel that the therapist is blaming them. It could be that patients perceive the focus on their contribution to the negative interaction cycle as blame.

The work related to decentering Janet's perspective, as spelled out previously, may be understood as explicit work on some problematic content, which may be premature for Janet if the problems on the process and relationship levels remain unaddressed. Although it is ultimately productive to work on changing problematic content, one could argue that other therapeutic work is needed before this. Beforehand, the therapist would have to clarify what type of relationship messages Janet needs to feel safe with the therapist and be able to trust them (one option may be the motive-oriented therapeutic relationship).

Another issue is related to Janet's hostility (in the relationship with family members), which may paradoxically lead to people leaving her, as a dramatic self-fulling prophecy. Her fear is confirmed, and people reject her because she is expressing this hostility. Before she even knows what content she has to work on (i.e., her schematic assumptions driving her interpersonal behaviors), it may be important for Janet to be aware of her part in her problematic social interactions. Raising her awareness of what she contributes through her behavior may increase her curiosity about what could make her behave in that way and not in another (i.e., her experiences, convictions, schematic assumptions). This may then increase her awareness that she will be able to choose herself and, ultimately, be motivated to clarify what is happening to codetermine her behavior.

"I Have Nobody. I'd Rather Die": Addressing the Patient's Sense of Not Belonging

In the following therapy session, Janet presented as extremely depressed and hopeless. She sobbed uncontrollably throughout the session, and it was difficult to engage her in any productive dialogue. Amidst her sobbing, she repeatedly stated,

> I'm all alone; I'm completely alone. I have nobody. I don't have the ability to change anything, and I don't want to go through life on my own with nobody to help me. I'd rather die.

Dialectical Behavior Perspective: Increasing Awareness and Tolerance of Aversive Emotions

In this session, Janet is clearly grappling with a profound sense of aloneness and a feeling of not belonging. Her ongoing emotional dysregulation creates a barrier between her and the therapist, making it challenging to effectively engage in therapeutic work. To address this, the therapist can validate Janet's experience of loneliness as a means of reducing her emotional arousal. Validating statements can focus on normalizing her sense of aloneness, particularly in the context of her history of relational trauma.

The primary goal of therapy is to help Janet eliminate dysfunctional behaviors that hinder her personal growth. This involves increasing her awareness, tolerance, and acceptance of the underlying aversive emotions that drive her "escape behaviors." As long as she remains preoccupied with avoiding her emotions, these primary aversive emotions will continue to be feared, and the valuable information contained within them will remain unprocessed, preventing new learning from taking place.

A major strategy for facilitating awareness, acceptance, and transformation of primary emotional experiences is informal and formal exposure to emotions. Emotional exposure can be conducted both in-session and outside of therapy. For instance, during a session, the therapist can intervene by blocking Janet's judgmental narrative and constant crying because these behaviors likely perpetuate her avoidance of vulnerable emotions. The therapist might highlight the patient's judgments and help her communicate without self-judgment. To disrupt the patient's continual crying, the therapist could adopt an irreverent stance by sitting back, withdrawing, appearing disinterested, and saying to the patient, "Let me know when you're ready."

If the therapist can successfully engage the patient in productive thera-peutic work and dialogue, it becomes essential to address the problematic behaviors that occur outside of therapy sessions and contribute to her emo-tional avoidance and distress. This may involve working on reducing heavy drinking, anger outbursts, and excessive work hours.

By targeting both in-session and out-of-session behaviors, the therapist can help the patient break free from the cycle of emotional avoidance, enabling her to develop healthier coping strategies and achieve her therapeutic goals.

Building tolerance for such an emotional state would entail the ability to experience it without resorting to heavy drinking or excessive work on weekends. It involves learning how to sit with the difficulty and pain of this emotional experience rather than escaping from it through unhealthy coping mechanisms. The focus is on staying present with the emotions and not avoiding them.

Transforming the emotional state requires actively working to shift the intense experience of loneliness. This can be achieved through exposure, which provides an opportunity to fully engage with and experience this state. Through exposure, Janet can recognize how this emotional state becomes activated in her daily life, particularly as a result of her childhood experiences.

Transforming also involves helping Janet understand that this recurring emotional state is not a reflection of her being alone in the world. It requires her to recognize that she can cope with the negative state and the associated emotions and thoughts. The therapeutic process aims to support her in realiz-ing she is not alone and in developing the skills to manage and navigate these challenging emotional experiences effectively.

An important aspect of Janet's experience is her deeply ingrained percep-tion that she does not belong and is alone. This narrative can be understood as a result of repeated invalidating experiences that left her with overwhelming and unmanageable painful emotions. Blaming herself became a coping strat-egy that provided a sense of control in the face of these challenging emotions. However, this self-perception of not belonging significantly influences her behavior and interactions with others.

It is crucial to assist Janet in recognizing that her experience of "alone-ness" and the belief that she does not belong are subjective states that can be shifted. These perceptions contribute to her aggressive posture, avoidance of social interactions, and fear of engaging with others. The therapist's role is to support her in challenging and transforming this self-view.

The therapist can help shift Janet's self-perception by guiding her to identify and validate her thoughts within the context of her personal history and learning experiences. By exploring the connection between her thoughts, mood, and behaviors, the therapist can assist her in recognizing the impact of her self-narrative on her overall well-being. The therapeutic process may involve encouraging Janet to act in ways that are opposite to her negative self-views, thereby challenging the validity of those views.

Ultimately, the goal is to help Janet develop a more balanced and accurate view of herself. This entails recognizing that her self-narrative is not an absolute truth and can be reshaped through therapeutic exploration and practice. By shifting her perception of herself, Janet can begin to engage with others in a less defensive and fearful manner, fostering more fulfilling and authentic social interactions.

Emotion-Focused Perspective: Emotional Experiences and Secondary Processes

From an emotion-focused therapy (EFT) perspective, it makes sense that social interaction problems in Janet's case are reflected by her emotions. Her emotional experiences are not only the expression of hostility but also the multiple self-protective processes that result in avoidance of emotions. It seems important to understand these processes as the possible consequences of her traumatic experience when she was little. An experiential therapist would probably add to this elaboration that exposure to this loneliness through a series of interventions may not be enough to provide a deep transformative experience. Here, the aim would be to change emotion with emotion, as Leslie Greenberg (2019) put it. The idea is to activate the emotion but not aim at a habitual effect and be exposed to the emotion in a counterconditioning paradigm. The goal is for Janet to be in the emotion, arrive at it, accept it, and fully allow it. She would then be able to extract new information to have another type of experience that synthesizes the old emotion and this current experience. By being aware of how she felt when she was alone, she may realize she needed somebody to comfort her or reach out to her and say, "Look, you're not alone." This process of repairing the wound where the original trauma happened will probably be an important step along the way.

There may be a distinction between what an EFT approach focuses on and an emotional exposure approach. While there may be differences, the overlaps are more convincing: Emotional exposure does involve accessing new emotional information. Therefore, the transformation of the emotional experience comes about through awareness of new information and new learning that occurs through the process of fully experiencing the avoided emotion. Unlike EFT, it may also be helpful to see emotional exposure as a form of transformation of emotion through new emotional information.

From a clarification-oriented viewpoint, one would assume that Janet's perception or fear of what is going to happen or not happen are probably aspects of more secondary reactions to her core loneliness. It may be interesting to consider these momentary movements within the patient, such as when the patient is approaching her core issues in psychotherapy. Chances are high (irrespective of the therapeutic relationship and specific motivation to change) that the experience of ambivalence toward this core loneliness will increase. A patient who expresses this perception or fear may be the norm, so Janet may say, "Look, I've tried so hard. So many times, I had so many hopes in other therapists. I'm not gonna try once more. It's not worth trying!" This may be understood as the to-be-expected move toward the content periphery. Janet may bump back into more secondary, probably also potentially external (vs. internal) content oriented toward the therapist (including potential therapeutic ruptures) or also into socially problematic interactions. Such momentary perceptions and fears are the norm when patients like Janet approach their core traumatic loneliness in therapy. One thing therapists can do is be aware of these different aspects and go with the momentary movement into the external perspective (i.e., the secondary elements), but then also gently guide the patient using process guidance back to their primary core issues. If Janet was to remain stuck in this cycle, the therapist may offer metacommunication and describe and clarify this cycle explicitly as it is occurring, with the aim of raising awareness about it in the patient.

Transference-Focused Perspective: Therapeutic Presence and Fear of Closeness

From a transference-focused perspective, one would focus on the exposure mostly within the session though not necessarily exclusively. The therapist can counter the loneliness by being present. Because she might feel alone vis-à-vis the therapist in the session, the therapist can reality-test Janet's perception and reactions and what they might do to increase the loneliness. The latter may involve the patient not being forthcoming or withholding content; this is the kind of information a TFP therapist would look for. One would value what happens in the session as informative and as the focus because it can be discussed between the therapist and patient. We would call this an emotional exposure.

One additional point is worth mentioning in the context of Janet. She experiences loneliness and talks about it as if it is immutable, a belief she might have come to honestly. All three of us would disagree with this belief, as might others. Janet may experience some of what is suggested as invalidating her experience of feeling alone. And she might not necessarily find it convincing at a hypothetical level. Some patients may foreclose on hope because it is harder to hope for something and then be disappointed than to just foreclose on it and have some control over the fact that you are alone and accept it. Janet may have a strong motivation to want to feel lonely. It is almost as if she is sentenced to feeling lonely. In this case, it might even be harder to imagine that there is a chance Janet would not be lonely because any delay or failure in achieving that would make the loneliness that much more intense. In other words, if you desire something and do not get it, it hurts a lot, but if you allow yourself to say, "It is futile, and I do not desire it," it may not feel as hurtful, and you may also feel as if you have some control over it. If you feel, "I don't need that anyway," like the defensive reaction we may see in Janet, you pull away, avoid, and do not allow certain feelings. In psychodynamic terms, you do not believe your libidinal impulse or the desire for that closeness can be met.

Therapists cannot simply reassure the patient because they cannot guarantee that the patient will find a partner and in what time frame. Although Janet may feel some emotional closeness to the therapist in session, reinforcing the idea that the therapist can offer some closeness and that this is possible, it might stoke fear in Janet about the close relationship and the fact that this therapeutic relationship is an artificial relationship—therapists do not typically think about their patients on Friday nights. The activation of feeling close, together with fear, may then result in the patient pulling back.

TFP is a nonjudgmental stance that allows people to talk about the thoughts and feelings that come into mind, even those that seem unacceptable or contradictory, which are important to figuring out what might be happening. It is important to walk a line between helping patients talk about difficult things and, at the same time, not imposing a preconceived structure that might feel invalidating to them.

For example, facing someone who lost a relationship, one might say—although it is a cliché—"There are other fish in the sea." Although it is a common thing people say to somebody when a relationship breaks up, it is usually experienced as unsupportive and invalidating. TFP would solve the dilemma by offering a nonjudgmental stance and trying not to either reinforce the distortion that this person will be lonely forever or invalidate a feeling that seems legitimate to them because they have been lonely for 40 years and cannot envision what it is that therapists might envision for them. Such patients do not necessarily know what a better world would look like.

The bottom line may be that the hopefulness of therapy is the promise of a better life, even though the patient, having gotten much better, cannot necessarily see making the next leap and genuinely doubts it is possible.

In extremis, a patient may see a therapist as someone who was corrupt and promised a duplicitous bill of sale. Janet will need increased capacity to be able to deal with these dilemmas.

"Why Are You the Only Therapist Who Doesn't Have a White Noise Machine?": Addressing In-Session Complaints

Janet frequently began sessions with subtle complaints about the therapist. In one session, she entered the therapy office and stated in a tone of annoyance,

> Why are you the only therapist who doesn't have a white noise machine? Every counseling office I've seen has white noise machines.

Within the broader functional domain of problematic social interaction, how does the therapist address the patient's perception that the therapist is uncaring and unsupportive when ruptures arise in the therapy relationship?

Plan Analysis Perspective: Complaints as Forms of Control

Janet's statement may be understood as part of her interpersonal pattern of avoidance of her inner experience and a way of turning her focus externally, seeking to put the fault on contextual issues, particularly the person of the therapist (thus making it a problem on the level of the relationship, as specified previously). On the basis of the case description, one could speculate that Janet has an activated plan of presenting as somebody who is asking something particular or needs to show that she is mindful of how therapy works. A white noise machine is not something people are generally familiar with; highlighting this detail may have an instrumental component in the current therapeutic relationship and reveal a problematic social interaction pattern. With this particular issue, Janet shows that she knows a lot about privacy issues in therapy. This may be a way of controlling the therapy relationship, which may not be helpful but is part of her more stable interpersonal style. These plans may serve the unproblematic aims of feeling protected and avoiding being hurt.

The therapist could address this situation using a motive-oriented therapeutic intervention either before this sequence or as part of an alliance rupture resolution strategy. When the therapist addresses such an externally focused move by the patient, they can make explicit how important it is to give Janet a particularly good therapy or something helpful to her in a safe environment. The therapist may directly show Janet that they are willing to take an extra step with her to provide safety (within the boundaries of the therapeutic relationship), which seems important at this point. This could involve saying something like, "It's so important for me that you notice all these details that show how important it is for you to have a safe relationship with me, and you know there's no information going out of this room. You seem to know quite a bit about how psychotherapy works, and I want to listen to you as best I can to make that space particularly safe for you." At this point, the therapist would avoid answering a specific content question (although it may be useful to answer them later) but would make a general—and genuine—comment about Janet's knowledge and competency in therapy. The idea is to build on Janet's specific resources to construct a positive and trustworthy therapeutic relationship.

Dialectical Behavior Perspective: Complaints as Secondary Emotional Responses

Janet's response can be seen as another instance of her tendency to perceive others as being neglectful of her needs and not being there for her. It is possible that she harbors a fear of trusting others, leading her to be hypervigilant in observing how they may fall short in being responsive and protective of her. In this case, her expectation was that a therapist would prioritize her privacy by using a white noise machine, and she feels let down by her therapist's failure to do so. This perception aligns with a recurring belief she holds about herself in relation to others: "I'm always being let down by others who aren't there for me." The absence of the white noise machine likely triggers deeper feelings of mistrust, evoking emotions such as fear, pain, and a profound sense of aloneness.

The clinical challenge lies in how to address these ruptures in the therapeutic alliance, particularly if they occur frequently during sessions. It may not be productive to directly explore each subtle attack on the alliance because doing so might shift the focus of the discussion solely onto relationship problems, potentially derailing the development of positive experiences within the therapeutic alliance. Timing is also crucial because delving into this dysfunctional perception within the context of the therapy relationship too early may be emotionally overwhelming. It is important for the therapeutic relationship to maintain a balance and not be dominated by discussions solely focused on relationship problems. A light comment in response to the patient's concern can be effective in repairing the therapeutic alliance. The therapist may offer validation by acknowledging Janet's perception and reassuring her that the therapy space is safe. For instance, the therapist could say, "I want to assure you that this is a safe space, and I apologize if not having a white noise machine made you feel like I don't value your privacy."

In addition, if the therapist has noticed a recurring pattern in Janet's tendency to view others as unsupportive, it can be helpful to bring awareness to this pattern. The therapist may gently point out the patient's familiar worry thought by saying, "When you made that comment, I noticed a recurring thought coming up for you: 'People aren't looking out for me.' Are you aware of that thought?"

By addressing Janet's concerns and highlighting any recurring patterns of negative thinking, the therapist can foster a sense of safety and encourage self-reflection, ultimately supporting the therapeutic process.

Transference-Focused Perspective: Repairing the Rupture While Fostering Trust

It would be helpful to have a balance between focusing on the potential rupture and the necessity of fostering trust in the relationship. However, if the core issue in this current rupture is not addressed, it will fester. Obviously, there is some level of distrust. When the therapist shows that they can talk about it in a matter-of-fact, reflective, serious way, they model for the patient the fact that things can be talked about, and when they avoid it, they implicitly reinforce the idea that things are dangerous and cannot be discussed.

SUMMARY: HOW TO MOVE TOWARD INTERPERSONAL EFFECTIVENESS

This chapter explored different therapeutic approaches to treating patients with personality disorders who exhibit disturbances in the functional domain of interpersonal and social functioning. We began by reviewing the empirical evidence for bringing about therapeutic change in the domain of social functioning, followed by the case study of a patient exhibiting severe interpersonal distress and poor social functioning. We then compared our different theoretical formulations of this case through an informal discussion and described our interventions in response to specific moments in therapy sessions, using the patient's verbatim statements as the starting points or opportunities for change.

With regard to empirical evidence, we reviewed the relationship between changes in interpersonal and social constructs and treatment outcome. Research findings mostly support the theory that changes in constructs related to social cognitive processing, including reflective functioning, mentalization, interpersonal patterns and cognitions, and theory of mind, are associated with positive outcomes (Kramer et al., 2020). However, there is a lack of research on how the use of specific interventions accounts for treatment effects. It also appears that these general constructs, measured globally across sessions, seem abstract in the light of an individual case requiring moment-by-moment assessments of the patient's interpersonal awareness and competence to implement a responsive intervention.

In our discussion of the case of Janet, a range of interventions were recommended. We identified several common change processes as important: validation of the patient's perspective, helping Janet reflect on her perceptions, helping her become curious and open to alternative perceptions, focusing on the underlying motives, applying relational strategies to minimize ruptures in the therapeutic alliance, strategically using interpretations when such ruptures arise (see also Chapter 9), and helping Janet express her needs. These themes are expanded on next.

When patients present in therapy with extremely irrational thoughts about interactions and recurring maladaptive interpersonal problems, it may be important to maintain an open, nonjudgmental, and accepting stance. The therapist should begin by carefully listening, seeking to understand, empathizing, and validating what makes sense from patients' perspectives. This includes understanding and appreciating how patients' perceptions may be understood in terms of their past circumstances and a sound case formulation.

In the context of activated problematic social interaction, we recommend that therapists avoid moving in too quickly to challenge patients' perceptions. Instead, encouraging patients to become curious about their perceptions may be most useful. Differentiating patients' content from their quality of processing and relationship (with the therapist) and focusing on the latter two before the former may help disentangle some of the activated problems. Facilitating insight requires openness and a demonstration of interest in understanding patients' perceptions. It is usually most productive to focus on specific, concrete examples of interpersonal interactions and explore them through an emotionally engaged dialogue to help patients consider which aspects of a story make sense and which may have entailed assumptions. Validation, clarification, redirection, and highlighting, in addition to the motive-oriented therapeutic relationship, are especially useful for promoting this type of reflection. In addition to clarification processes, certain therapy approaches also use interpretations to increase the precision of patients' representational systems, potentially leading to lasting change.

The focus on validating patients' recurring maladaptive perceptions of social interactions has to be balanced with a focus on changing or challenging them. One task is to help patients recognize how their maladaptive perceptions are part of a broader pattern and arise in multiple situations. Another is to gently challenge patients by helping them consider alternative perceptions, either by offering an interpretation or by using self-disclosure to convey another point of view. It can also be beneficial to help patients understand how their perceptions may be contributing to their emotions, interpersonal behaviors, and thoughts. For example, when Janet thinks she will be rejected by others, how does it influence her behaviors with them? Ideally, psychotherapy research should increasingly study change on these detailed and clinically relevant levels and their moment-by-moment changes rather than on generic markers associated with problematic social patterns.

In therapy, patients can also be helped to address the emotional needs that underlie their perceptions, with the aim of transforming maladaptive emotional experiences. Rather than intervening at the level of an expressed (social-cognitive) statement, the therapist can respond to the emotional need underlying that statement. This may foster some relief in the patient and a feeling of being understood if the relational need is satisfied (see Chapter 4). The next step may entail helping patients gain more awareness, generate more effective ways to communicate, and address these needs in relationships in their daily lives.

Developing a positive therapy alliance is arguably essential, but maintaining it can be challenging when working with patients whose problems are dominated by high levels of mistrust and interpersonal and social difficulties. To avoid precipitating a breakdown in the alliance, therapists should always respond with high levels of support and validation and refrain from being confrontational or prematurely offering interpretations of irrational perceptions. Nurturing a positive alliance also requires closely monitoring one's reactions to avoid being (unhelpfully) reactive. It is important to maintain a compassionate and empathic stance because understanding patients' difficulties within their context is an antidote to negative judgments.

With patients who are highly sensitive to interpersonal threats, minor or major ruptures and breakdowns in the therapeutic alliance will inevitably arise, and when they do, they must be addressed with sensitivity (see Chapter 9). Even when therapists try their best to be sufficiently supportive and validating, the therapy process can entail frequent and persistent ruptures, and it is neither productive nor feasible to address each one. It may be important for the therapist to focus on the underlying motive and validate it instead of the apparent behavior in the room. However, if a rupture is prominent, it should be repaired directly and explicitly. It is important not to become (unhelpfully) reactive but to remain empathic and develop an empathic understanding of the patient's response. Interventions that can be useful for navigating ruptures include attunement to and validation of the patient's underlying needs and motives, an exploration of the patient's experience, and acknowledgment of possibly having contributed to the rupture oneself. Therapists could help patients observe what triggered the rupture, explore their experience of it, and, if appropriate, link the rupture to broader dysfunctional interpersonal patterns, including early formative relationships with others. The case formulation can be used to anticipate the triggers for ruptures so that they do not arise out of the blue and can be prevented. It is important to pay attention to subtle indicators of a rupture—for example, Janet's complaint about her therapist's lack of a white noise machine.

In sum, what is common to each of our perspectives is the importance of using supportive strategies to cultivate a positive therapeutic relationship, including careful listening, validating, and maintaining an open and curious stance. Together with clarification and interpretation, these may deepen patients' awareness of their problematic social interaction patterns and help them learn how to dissolve and overcome them. Ruptures in the therapeutic alliance are inevitable, and we emphasize the importance of choosing the best timing to address these when they arise. Whatever the therapeutic approach, the end goals are to help patients to understand their perceptions of social interaction, observe their impact, become aware of recurring problematic perceptions, shift from undifferentiated rigid perceptions to a more nuanced way of viewing themselves and others, and move toward more interpersonal effectiveness.

6 MOVING FROM IDENTITY DIFFUSION TO AN INTEGRATED SENSE OF SELF

This chapter explores changes in the functional domain of identity disturbance in patients with personality pathology. *Identity* is a multifaceted construct and broadly refers to an individual's representations of self and others, their values, and role commitments (Westen, 1985). Identity is also referred to as the self, as in self-concept, and personality. Facets of identity include coherence; consistency in thoughts, feelings, and behaviors over time and situations; commitment to values and goals; appreciation of sameness across time; and a sense of boundary with others. The developers of the *Diagnostic and Statistical Manual of Mental Disorders* (5th ed., text rev.; American Psychiatric Association, 2022) and other theorists (Erikson, 1950; Kernberg, 1967) characterize a healthy sense of self as an intact or consolidated identity. People with a consolidated and intact sense of self typically experience themselves as unique, have a coherent sense of self across time and history, have a stable and accurate appraisal of themselves, and have clear boundaries between themselves and others. Self-esteem is realistic and resilient to challenges in a healthy individual. In addition, compared with individuals with a diffuse sense of self, individuals with intact identities experience greater capacity for

https://doi.org/10.1037/0000388-007
Understanding Mechanisms of Change in Psychotherapies for Personality Disorders, by U. Kramer, K. N. Levy, and S. McMain

a broad range of emotions and adaptive emotion-regulation capacities. Individuals with an intact sense of self have a greater capacity for self-direction and reflective decision making. People with an intact sense of self are especially better equipped than those with a diffuse sense of self to pursue coherent and meaningful short-term and long-term goals, maintain constructive relationships, and engage in prosocial standards of behavior.

Patients diagnosed with personality disorders can be distinguished by identity problems, and this may especially be true for those diagnosed with borderline personality disorder (BPD), who are typically distinguished by an identity diffusion. *Identity diffusion* is characterized by a lack of stability in past and present representations of self, uncertainty about self and fluctuating feelings about self, and a lack of cohesive identity. People with diffuse identities are prone to periods of excessive self-criticism, the externalization of problems, chronic feelings of emptiness, and transient feelings of dissociation in times of stress or conflict. Frequent vacillations in identity and disparate representations of self interfere with the identification of goals, values, aspirations, and engagement in planful behavior. Identity problems also contribute to unstable interpersonal relationships. In contrast to those with BPD, people with narcissistic personality traits or disorder may have a more intact sense of self, although it may be pathologically grandiose at times as compensation for a more fragile sense of self.

Identity problems can manifest in several ways in treatment and can be difficult to change. When patients vacillate in their representation of themselves and others, therapists can react with confusion. In one moment, a therapist may respond to one presentation of self, leaving the patient feeling misunderstood and invalidated and the therapist confused as to why. Identity problems interfere with an individual's capacity to self-reflect and access and represent internal experience.

In this chapter, we consider how therapists may foster an integrated sense of self in patients with personality disorders. We first summarize the empirical support for the role of identity as a mechanism of change in the treatment of personality pathology. Our case discussion focuses on Leon, a man whose treatment was marked by a focus on his identity difficulties.[1] We examine how patients can move from identity diffusion to an integrated sense of self. We end the chapter with a summary statement on how the consolidation of identity can be understood as a mechanism of change in treatments of personality disorders.

---

[1]The case of Leon has been modified to disguise the patient's identity and protect their confidentiality.

EMPIRICAL SUPPORT FOR CONSOLIDATION IN IDENTITY AS A MECHANISM OF CHANGE

Of the domains identified as a process of change linked to outcomes, identity disturbance has received considerably little attention in psychotherapy research. No studies have directly examined whether change in identity disturbance is a mechanism of change. The following three studies are relevant to the clinical theory that consolidation in identity is a central mechanism in psychotherapy change. Scala et al. (2018) examined the relationship between self-concept clarity—a characteristic of identity problems—negative affect, and suicidal and self-injurious urges in 55 individuals with BPD. The findings showed that although negative affect and self-concept clarity did not predict self-injurious urges independently, there was a trend-level effect indicating negative affect and self-concept clarity predicted self-injurious urges. More specifically, when self-concept clarity was high, self-injurious urges were lower, even when negative affect was high.

In another study, Levy et al. (2006) found that changes in mentalizing and coherence of attachment narratives were associated with outcomes in transference-focused psychotherapy but not in dialectical behavior therapy (DBT) or supportive therapy. Mentalizing and coherence of attachment narratives, because they are representational constructs involving self and other representations, have been conceptualized as a proxy for identity. Incoherent narratives are similar to Kernberg's (2005) concept of identity diffusion; likewise, coherent narratives and high levels of mentalizing may reflect identity consolidation.

In a secondary analysis, Levy and colleagues (2010) found that vacillations of these mental states associated with the self-representations predicted problems in the patient–therapist alliance. Later work on the same sample found that specific techniques targeted to identity integration were associated with changes in mentalizing and attachment coherence (Kivity et al., 2019, 2021). The finding that identity, as measured by mentalization and coherence of attachment narratives, is linked to positive outcomes has been replicated in other studies (Bedics et al., 2012; Buchheim & George, 2011; Fischer-Kern et al., 2015; Levy et al., 2022).

THE CASE OF LEON

Leon is a 35-year-old cisgender man who identifies as heterosexual and is married with two children. He is unemployed though wealthy due to his father's support. He previously owned a company and was an investor in several businesses. His business ventures were all unprofitable, although they allowed him to portray himself to others as successful. He presented to treatment after his wife threatened him with a divorce because of his frequent angry outbursts at home and with others. During these outbursts, his behavior is extremely dysregulated; he has cursed and threatened others and threatened and damaged property. His wife reported that his anger outbursts scare people. His outbursts have occurred in public, leading to him being banned from various businesses. On several occasions, the police have been called due to his angry behavior. Although Leon describes himself as brilliant and talented, he recognizes that he is generally irritable and unhappy. He is in constant need of attention, recognition, and aggrandization and is quickly hurt or injured when he feels unrecognized for his abilities. When he presented to therapy, he could not function at work or in his capacity as a parent. Leon likened his wife and children to "a ball and chain" and blamed them for holding him back from being successful. He smokes marijuana daily to soothe his feelings of agitation.

Leon's identity disturbance is manifested in several ways. Despite his superior intelligence and artistic and technical abilities, he lacked direction and the ability to commit to activities and goals. His occupational and personal interests vacillated and contributed to his occupational dysfunction. Leon graduated from a prestigious college with a strong education. He is somewhat of a self-made polymath because he is knowledgeable about history, philosophy, political science, and classics and is confident in his knowledge. Upon graduation, with the help of his parents, he was offered and accepted a job at a prestigious political think tank. This is the only paid job he has had since his graduation. It was unclear whether he quit or was asked to leave the job. Leon explained that he was disillusioned by the mission of the organization. He was intolerant of the imperfections in others. He described his coworkers and bosses as hypocrites. He was intolerant of critical feedback and frequently perceived disapproval from others. He reported he did not like doing "grunt work" and believed his ideas were better than others'; he was upset that his talent was not recognized. Fed up with his treatment by others, he quit his job and went to Europe to reportedly "make it big." He returned to the United States relatively soon afterward and quickly married a woman he met in Europe and did not know particularly well, but he liked the idea of being married and thought it would please his parents.

Although he reported no interest in business throughout his life—he resented his father's business success and his neglect of Leon—he yearned to be successful, and despite little education in the area, he came to see business as a route to the recognition he sought. He fancied himself as an entrepreneur and invested in several business opportunities. He resented his business partners because he believed they did not value his advice and used him for his money. He frequently wished he had a different life and said that he would make different choices though he remained uncertain about what different path he would take. He frequently thought about buying out his partners and doing something different with the businesses. At other times, he had thoughts of leaving his partners, starting up his own competitive business, and running his partners into bankruptcy. Occasionally, he wished he had stayed in Europe and become a success overseas. His fantasies ranged across several different and disparate pursuits, and he flipped between his fantasies of success. He also thought of being a physician but was unwilling to take any prerequisite courses. He aspired to become a famous musician despite not knowing how to play a musical instrument. He wanted to be an international playboy. Still, at other times, he disparaged any ideas about what career path to pursue.

When he entered treatment, he had little direction and was unprepared to embark on a productive career path. In comparison to his peers, who had invested in training or education, gained expertise, and were ready to reap the benefits of their efforts in the form of promotion and job or business security, Leon floundered. He presented more like a recent college graduate who was considering his career options than as a 35-year-old person with a family. He resented the idea of paying his dues and instead wanted to be in charge at the outset of any career. He lamented that others did not recognize his talents and abilities. Despite being married with children, he derived little pleasure from family life. He frequently talked about the young high school women who had rejected him, and he lamented not going to his prom or pursuing these other relationships.

His identity diffusion showed itself in the therapy sessions, where he was difficult to follow because, at one moment, he would state he felt one way, and the next moment he felt something completely different. His mood and thoughts about himself and others rapidly changed. Sometimes his vacillations in mental states were minor. For example, during the initial assessment, he declared he has no friends: "I have no friends! No one. No one I can hang out with, no one I can call. It sucks." Later in the same session, he described spending time with friends and elaborated on several get-togethers. He described conversations with friends and referred to one individual as a good friend. At one point in this session, the therapist attempted to confront Leon with this discrepancy in his description of his friends, and he reacted angrily: "I never said that! Of course, I have friends—good friends to boot!" He shook his head in disbelief and disgust as if he could never present himself so inconsistently; he had little insight into his presentation.

Although his parents financially supported him, Leon was estranged from them, especially his father. He rarely saw his parents and only contacted them when he needed money. Leon spent many sessions complaining about his father and the stupid things he said and did. Despite his father's financial success and support, Leon was frequently highly dismissive of his father's business acumen. His derogatory comments about his father were occasionally extremely harsh; he referred to him as a "bug, an insect" who should be "squashed" or someone who could be "stepped on."

Despite devaluing his father, he yearned for his approval and admiration. On one occasion—on Father's Day—Leon's father invited him out for the day. Leon presented to session in an upbeat mood and excitedly told his therapist about the conversation and plans with his father. He praised his father for being a wonderful man and described him as a self-made business genius. This positive portrayal of his father starkly contrasted with his previous complaints about his father and the description of him as an idiot who had been lucky in business. His idealization of his father continued until Father's Day when his father called him early that morning and canceled their plans. According to Leon, his father had not elaborated and had been abrupt, gruff, and defensive. Leon did not know why his father canceled the plans, and the situation prompted an angry outburst from Leon. He destroyed several of his possessions, and the property damage was extensive and costly.

His wife contacted the therapist because Leon was also talking about killing himself. The therapist spoke to Leon, although they had difficulty assessing his suicide risk. In Leon's moments of calm, the therapist could respond supportively and ask him direct questions about his suicidal thoughts. At other moments, he escalated quickly into angry rants about his father. He stated that his father was "rotten," "the devil," "evil," and "the worst—worse than Hitler." It was evident that Leon was angry and hurt, and the therapist attempted to validate Leon while simultaneously trying to avoid reinforcing any distorted and extreme thoughts about his father. Leon's angry ranting was uncontainable, and it was hard for the therapist to help Leon modulate his anger. The therapist engaged in a gentle and empathic discussion, highlighting how disappointed Leon must have felt about his father canceling the plans. Rejecting the therapist's attempt to validate underlying feelings of hurt, Leon declared he was not disappointed: "Why would I be disappointed?" He continued to harshly criticize his father and maintain that he was a "bug, an insect that should be squashed." Leon declared he would never see his father again. He revealed a hint of his longing and disappointment when he declared it was his father who would be upset. Calm moments were short-lived, and he quickly escalated into anger. In a premature move, the therapist attempted to dissipate Leon's anger by highlighting Leon's disappointment and his desire to spend time with his father. This move prompted an increase in anger, and uncharacteristically, Leon screamed at his therapist, "I never said that!"

Over the course of the treatment, there were other dramatic signs of Leon's identity disturbance that manifested in extreme and shifting views of himself. As a child into his late teens, he described himself as a devout Christian, and he had a close relationship with the minister of his church. He was well-versed in the bible and religious script. At the same time, Leon presented himself as a staunch atheist. He was derogatory of others who were religious and scoffed at people who were spiritual, referring to them as mentally inferior. Despite his strong opinions about religion, he was drawn to women who were religious. At times, he criticized them, and at other times, engaged with them with ease in religious rituals and routines. At one point, he joined a new-age spiritual group, and despite a considerable investment of time and money in this community, he left after an argument with one of the spiritual leaders and returned to staunch atheist beliefs. This position contrasted with a fantasy he shared about wanting to start his own religion or cult that would destroy the group he had been engaged with. His ideas seemed so extreme that his therapist considered whether he was moving into a manic state or episode. Instead, Leon was merely having a narcissistic fantasy. A few years later, his interest in religion was renewed, and he thought of becoming a clergyman or a theologian. Leon showed no awareness of how he rapidly vacillated between different ideals for himself.

In the next section, we turn to our case formulation to understand how to make sense of this clinical material.

CASE FORMULATION: UNDERSTANDING IDENTITY DISTURBANCE

Case formulation is a basis for understanding Leon's identity disturbances. We begin by conceptualizing Leon's identity disturbance from our three perspectives and then propose a synthesized formulation.

Plan Analysis Formulation: Find Common Ground in the Patient's Accomplishments

From a plan analysis perspective, this patient has a self-presentation that is oppositional in its content. On the one hand, this person presents as particularly intelligent and special, somebody for whom only the best is good enough. On the other hand, it seems he is not working toward greatness or intelligence but has had everything handed to him—his father helped him get his first job and supports him financially. From a plan analysis perspective, it may be helpful to consider the underlying motive for these conflicting self-presentations. Leon is motivated to be recognized as someone valuable or unique, but more observational data is needed to determine the details of the formulation. In such a context, the first thing a therapist would want to understand is how to welcome the idea that Leon may need a particularly good treatment, which may represent a first "common ground" with Leon. A therapist entering into a therapeutic relationship with Leon could assume that, by highlighting these opposing views, Leon would feel threatened or even have the urge to run away because he would not tolerate the confrontation. So the first idea may be to meet Leon at a "high level," noting that he has achieved quite a bit, despite some difficulties, and from there, finding more common ground. After arriving at this common ground, one could gently try to define a problematic area that could be improved with therapy. Focusing on the underlying motive may mean seeing what Leon has already accomplished.

What is striking in Leon's case is that he seems to fundamentally lack perspective; it is unclear where he is going in life. This may be underpinned by difficulties in identity and affect regulation, which may be explained by determining specific plans in the case formulation. It is clear that this patient, not knowing where he is going, may have the experience of "walking in the same spot," making it difficult to find common ground with the therapist (and potentially anyone else). What is the purpose of having this experience of lacking direction (one would ask from a plan analytic viewpoint)? It may serve a plan such as "avoid engaging fully in one direction or another," which may, again, serve some more fundamental plan related to avoidance of failure or the experience of being ineffective. All this may be related to some basic motive of self-preservation or control over his life, maintaining his relationship with his parents in some way, or regulating affect. The latter may be the most fundamental (and highest in the hierarchy of plans; see also Caspar, 2018 for a discussion of patients' fantasies in plan analysis). A possible plan involving the overarching motive of affect regulation may be "to avoid and escape from specific negative emotions." The case presentation shows that Leon never had the opportunity to ask himself, "Do I really want this?" So one could also hypothesize that he is alienated from his internal experience and lacks self-referential activity. This lack of connection with his innermost preference and needs connected with his primary adaptive emotions related to these issues should be addressed in therapy.

Dialectical Behavior Formulation: Understanding Environmental Factors

From a dialectical behavior perspective, it is crucial to understand Leon's identity disturbance within the context of his upbringing and the factors that influenced his sense of self. Specifically, his relationship with his parents sheds light on his identity struggles. Leon recalled numerous instances of invalidation from his parents, particularly his critical and distant father, as well as his emotionally unavailable mother. These pervasive experiences of invalidation likely contribute to Leon's fluctuating self-states, anger outbursts, and difficulties functioning effectively. They also point to a broader issue in his emotion regulation abilities.

Repeated dismissal and criticism have hindered Leon's ability to validate his emotional experiences. Individuals who have faced persistent invalidation often struggle to acknowledge, tolerate, and authentically experience their emotions, especially negative emotions. Leon has developed coping mechanisms such as judgmental behavior, anger outbursts, job avoidance, and quitting, all aimed at avoiding or escaping aversive emotions. However, this avoidance prevents him from learning how to modulate intense negative emotions effectively and inhibits the transformation of these emotions and his emotional growth.

Furthermore, the capacity for identity development relies on the ability to fully experience and express emotions, identify personal preferences, and communicate emotional needs. Leon faces challenges in directly expressing his emotional needs within his relationships. He compensates for this by projecting an image of extreme competence and success, aspiring to be a famous musician or physician, yet failing to take meaningful steps toward these careers. Leon's lofty expectations and pursuit of perfection may have been internalized by the repeated criticism he received from his father. Excessive criticism often prevents individuals from tolerating struggle, failure, and imperfection.

The absence of consistent and predictable emotional experiences also hinders the development of a stable sense of self. Leon's emotions appear volatile and unpredictable, potentially triggered by experiences of failure, which elicit profound feelings of shame. To cope with this shame, Leon adopts a grandiose and narcissistic presentation of himself. His frequent anger serves as an escape from underlying shame.

In DBT, a dialectical perspective acknowledges the interplay between Leon's sense of self and his perceptions of others. He struggles to form consistent and predictable views of himself and others, vacillating between extremely positive and negative judgments. Paradoxically, he judges himself and others equally. These judgments serve as a strategy that allows Leon to avoid the full experience of his emotions and access to information about his emotional needs and preferences. For instance, when his father cancels plans abruptly, Leon's immediate anger shields him from experiencing valid feelings of disappointment, and this prevents him from seeking self-soothing. His self-judgments have become a narrative that shapes his overall self-concept.

Transference-Focused Formulation: Conflicts in Self-Other Representations

From a transference-focused perspective, which is a bit different from an affect regulation perspective, it remains an open question how affect is related to identity disturbance. What is most relevant is Leon's sensitivity to slights. These are not necessarily criticisms where he is invalidated and put down. If Leon walks into a store and an employee does not walk up to him fast enough to ask if they can help him (because they are attending to something else or at the register with another customer), he could fly into a rage because he expects people to kowtow to him. Some of the perception of being criticized or invalidated is not concordant with his experiences.

At other times, Leon is painfully aware of how little he has accomplished and may not be able to accomplish what he wants to. As a result, he often vacillates between grandiose statements about his capacity, acumen, and ability to do things and avoidance of tasks and activities he is otherwise committed to. In addition, he had difficulty maintaining his commitment when he experienced the slightest bumps in the road, and he would quickly give up. These oscillations between grandiose self-representation and vulnerability can be viewed as part of identity disturbance as much as emotion dysregulation. Leon vacillates between self-aggrandizement and being aware of how little he has accomplished, externalizing those moments. For example, he may say his father did not teach him how to do things or he did not become a great athlete because of his father's lack of support.

His internal experience is often one of feeling insignificant and incapable and then vacillating to a puffed-up, exaggerated presentation that seems false. Contact with accomplished people may leave him feeling insignificant. What seems to be at the core of Leon's problems is his representations of himself and others, as well as his self-representations in relation to those of others and the emotional aspects of these representations. Identity disturbance may be an inconsistent picture of the self and experience of the other vis-à-vis the self that makes it hard for the person to act in a directed or coherent manner—in one moment, they represent themselves one way, and at another moment, they represent themselves in another way. There is both a cognitive and affective level to these representations. It is hard for patients who cannot regulate themselves well to have representations of themselves in a more coherent, goal-directed way. Likewise, it is hard for patients who cannot see themselves in a consistent way to regulate emotions.

Toward a Common Formulation

In a synthesis of our three case formulation perspectives, we see a tension between the more representational perspective on explaining identity issues, the more affect-oriented perspective, and the goal- or motive-oriented explanations of these issues. On the one hand, Leon's functioning may be seen as avoiding emotional experiences (primary emotions). On the other hand, one could conceive that he is not avoiding emotions because he is in the thralls of emotional experience in the here and now. That is, Leon is avoiding one set of emotions, but he finds himself at the mercy of another set of emotions. In addition, the tension between an affect-oriented explanation and a cognitive-oriented explanation of identity issues is also at play. One could argue that Leon is avoiding cognitive states, not just emotional states (i.e., his self-concept of being a failure). A DBT perspective may give precedence to the emotional aspects underlying the self-concept. Leon cannot adequately use his emotional experience to guide adaptive tendencies. From a transference-focused psychotherapy (TFP) perspective, representational aspects of the dynamic are at the forefront, though all representations have affect attached. Leon does not have an organized representational capacity that allows him to downregulate his emotions adequately. From a plan analysis case formulation perspective, the motives driving the self-presentation are the anchor.

What is common across all three perspectives is that irrespective of where we start from, all aspects are finally integrated into a coherent explanation focusing on the phenomenology of the case. We agree that certain experiences described by Leon must be particularly uncomfortable—even aversive—to him, making him suffer and come into therapy. An example of this is Leon being discombobulated and dysregulated. In addition, we agree that identity affects cognitive–affective motivationally grounded behaviors, such as Leon's presentation in session, his anger, and his not knowing what he wants to do for his career. We also agree that these behaviors have particular meanings in relationships (e.g., with his father and potentially with the therapist) and impact the quality of his view of others. There seems to be, for identity issues, a dynamic interplay between Leon's behaviors, emotional experiences, core motives, and representations of self and others, each impacting one another so the therapist could intervene at any level.

CHOICE POINTS AND OPPORTUNITIES FOR CHANGE

For the remainder of this chapter, we focus on two choice points from Leon's treatment selected for the themes in the case formulation and the topic of problematic identity disturbance. First, we consider a typical situation with Leon during which he presents diverse and contrasting representations of himself in session. At this juncture in the therapy, we consider how to help Leon develop a more integrated view of himself. The second choice point is a situation in which Leon presents with an extremely negative view of his father. At this juncture, we ask ourselves how to help Leon develop more differentiated representations of others. After discussing our intervention approaches, we conclude with a summary statement that synthesizes gained knowledge from our perspectives and relevant research that informs the patient's move toward an integrated sense of self as a potential mechanism of change in treatments for personality disorders. Table 6.1 synthesizes generic

TABLE 6.1. How to Foster a Path Toward an Integrated Sense of Self

Generic therapist interventions	Specific therapist interventions	Patient processes
Choice point: Addressing a disparate experience of the self		
• Clarify the therapy mission.	• Focus on the consequences.	• Be aware of one's contribution to the problem.
• Do a case formulation.	• Focus on the conflict.	• Be aware of conflict and precipitants.
• Provide contingent responsiveness.	• Express confusion.	
• Offer support and understanding.	• Validate the patient's confusion.	• Be aware of one's impact on others.
• Focus on change in confusion.	• Challenge perception.	• Feel welcome despite confusion.
• Use accessible language.	• Use metaphors and interpretation.	• Clarify confusion.
		• Build meaning.
		• Connect with the therapist and understand their confusion.
		• Learn to own the confusion.
Choice point: Addressing conflictual representations of the other		
• Focus on the here and now.	• Focus on emotional experience.	• Be aware of emotional reactions.
• Offer understanding.	• Focus on strengthening identity.	• Build on activated resources.
• Use accessible language.	• Validate the valid.	• Connect with the therapist and feel understood.
	• Use metaphors and interpretation.	• Understand confusion and dissolve it.

and approach-specific strategies that therapists might use, as well as relevant patient processes, in the two choice points presented in this chapter.

"No, I Did Not Say This!": Developing a More Integrated Sense of Experience

This brief excerpt reflects a typical scenario between Leon and his therapist. In response to the therapist's accurate reflection of Leon's experience, he erupted in anger and rejected the therapist's validation. How does a therapist address a patient's conflicting views of themselves? What does a therapist do to help a patient like Leon develop an integrated and coherent sense of themselves? When a patient is identity diffused, as in the case of Leon, they can experience themselves differently from one moment to the next. The patient can shift rapidly between different views of themselves. Patients like Leon can readily externalize their problems and blame others. A therapeutic challenge is to bring disowned aspects of the self into the patient's awareness. What complicates handling this clinical scenario is that confronting the patient with disowned or unacknowledged experiences may threaten the patient. At the same time, a therapist's failure to address the patient's discrepant views of the self can impede therapeutic progress. So, while it is essential to help the patient develop a more integrated sense of self, the issue is how to navigate this choice point skillfully so the therapist does not precipitate a major rupture in the therapeutic alliance.

Clarification-Oriented Perspective: Understand Where the Patient Is in the Therapy Process

From a clarification-oriented psychotherapy perspective—which directly builds on the earlier plan analysis formulation (Sachse, 2020)—the first question may be to know where Leon currently is in his therapy process. For now, we know that Leon seeks treatment. He said at one point, "I have no friends" and "This sucks," which expresses suffering. We then observed this opposing or inconsistent presentation of the self: He presented in one way, and then, when the therapist repeated what Leon said, he responded, "No, I didn't say that; you're making this up!" The therapist may have intended to bring these opposing, oscillating views about the self together and move in with this confrontation, but the patient did not follow suit.

It may be important to take a step back and ask oneself as a therapist where this patient is in this process. Does he know why he is coming to therapy and what he wants to get out of this process? What is he seeking here? What is he expecting? What would be helpful for him to know? What kind of insight would be necessary for him to move forward, and when? Is he motivated or ready to hear and process certain things (now or later)? Is he open?

From what we know, it may be hard for Leon, at this juncture in the psychotherapy, to consider that these opposing self-presentations are just two sides of the same coin. So when he said, "It sucks," and "I have no friends," one could assume that this (supposedly) authentic statement may be conceptualized as a negative consequence or "cost" of his problematic behavior, which he is completely unaware of at that point. It could be that, by adopting certain interaction styles, Leon is producing problematic behavior he does not want (which, therefore, produces the disparity and the feeling that "it sucks"). A clarification-oriented therapist would identify this dilemma as part of the specific therapy phase when the therapeutic mission (or overall tasks) must be agreed on (see Sachse, 2020). In this context, the therapist could give Leon feedback by gently saying (when he says he has no friends), "This is interesting. So you actually have no friends." This is to mark something that Leon does not seem to want, making it a potential focus of intervention or something Leon may want to change (now or later). To make this more explicit, the therapist may want to spend more time on this and slow down the process at this juncture. It means the therapist conveys understanding for a consensus that will not be disputed later in therapy. This may lay the ground for a focus on where to potentially have an effect with the therapy, implicitly conveying to the patient, "This is what we could work on if you decide to do so."

Without a clear case formulation, the therapist would not know which content to follow or focus on. If the patient is interested, this will point inward toward the patient's inner experience (rather than externally, to other people, and so forth). The aim of this particular intervention is for the patient to walk out of this session, saying to himself, "This is a problem that I am causing in my life. I am the one with the problematic schema or interaction problems that causes exactly what I fear the most or what I don't want. And this therapist can help me uncover it, get awareness of it, and resolve it." This is some of the groundwork of the therapeutic mission, which may pave the path toward a more integrated understanding of oneself (achieved with the help of the therapy).

Of course, once the patient reacts in the way shown in the transcript and denies what he said before, the therapist could also offer their confusion about it: "I am confused. Can you say more about what makes you react so strongly right now?" Again, this may lead to work on the therapeutic mission.

Dialectical Behavior Perspective: Building Awareness of Judgmental Thoughts

Patients like Leon who exhibit fluctuating and extreme views of themselves and others often engage in strong judgments, whether negative or positive. It is crucial to start by enhancing Leon's awareness of his thoughts regarding himself and others. Helping Leon observe and recognize his judgmental thoughts as they arise in the present moment is important. The therapist can assist Leon in identifying the recurring patterns and content of his self-judgments and judgments of others. In addition, it would be beneficial to help Leon identify the triggers, both internal and external, that elicit his judgmental thoughts. For instance, the therapist can guide Leon in recognizing the situational cues that provoke his grandiose self-views, such as thoughts of becoming a famous musician. This initial step of recognizing the underlying emotions avoided by his judgmental thoughts is crucial.

In DBT, various strategies can be employed to increase Leon's self-awareness, including his perceptions, thoughts, and emotions. The therapist can intervene by observing and highlighting Leon's emotions and thoughts. For example, if the therapist notices something they said has struck a nerve, they can acknowledge it by saying, "It seems like something I said has affected you deeply." If the patient responds with high levels of anxiety, defensiveness, or anger, as demonstrated by their confrontation ("No, I did not say this; you are making this up"), the therapist can validate their emotions in those moments. They might say, "It's understandable that you're upset with me if I've misunderstood you," or "I apologize if it feels uncomfortable that I saw it that way." However, it is important for the therapist to exercise caution and not inadvertently validate or endorse the patient's distorted views as reasonable or rational.

Next, the therapist can draw attention to the patient's recurring patterns of thoughts about themselves and others. For deeply ingrained beliefs, the therapist can explicitly orient the patient to the issue and bring it to their awareness. The therapist can intentionally emphasize the repetitive nature of the belief, for example, by saying, "Have you noticed that you frequently have thoughts that others are attacking you?" If Leon responds to this challenge with a sense of threat or heightened vulnerability, the therapist can provide validation before challenging the patient and assisting them in considering alternative ways of thinking and adopting a more dialectical perspective of themselves.

Transference-Focused Perspective: Slowly Unpack Avoidant Behaviors and Relationship Dynamics

From a TFP perspective, one would use slightly different language for describing similar processes. First, the therapist may want to determine whether the strategy used to avoid the affect is conscious. Doing so might require gentle questioning to clarify the patient's phenomenological experience in the moment. In the literature, scholars have distinguished between conscious coping styles and defense mechanisms, which in contrast, are conceptualized as being unconscious. Talking about unconscious processes too soon, before it is closer to the patient's awareness, can be jarring to patients and may not resonate with them at best, and they may feel attacked at worst. When a thought or a feeling is too disturbing to a patient, they may, using psychodynamic language, split it off (also known as the defense mechanism of splitting). From a more behavioral tradition, the language of experiential avoidance is used, but the concepts are similar (Hayes et al., 1996).

It may be arbitrary to define emotion or thought as primary, given that all thoughts have an affect attached, and all affects have a representation (Kernberg, 1982, 2006). For a patient, escaping aversive thoughts and feelings may be intertwined, and some of the process may be available to the patient for reflection, but some of the experience, at least at some times, may not be readily available and may need time to unpack. Two metaphors are useful for conceptualizing this process. The first is the concept of the bends in scuba diving. A diver has to return to the surface slowly; otherwise, the experience may be painful or even deadly. Bringing a split-off or avoided idea to the surface may take time and care. Similarly, the metaphor of cooking a stew comes to mind. Turning up the flame on the stove will not make the flavors of the stew coalesce any quicker. The stew may be hot enough to eat, but it will not have a rich flavor.

The person may feel closeness with the therapist, which might scare them because it brings up feelings of dependency and vulnerability. As a result, they may then react by pushing the therapist away. Coming late or not at all to session may be a reaction to feelings of dependency and the associated vulnerability. Likewise, "flights into health," where a patient precipitously "feels better" as a defense against the anxieties and/or depression associated with the therapy work, can lead them to want to end therapy. This can happen in the patient's life outside of therapy as well, in other close relationships with friends or significant others. Thus, the question arises as to whether these dynamics that play out with the therapist in the consultation room can be discussed and, if so, at what level of depth. Therapists have to be careful when discussing the patient's dependency on them because patients can understandably find such discussions make them feel vulnerable and even humiliated. It can be painful to want something from another, especially in a relationship like the therapeutic one with its strict professional boundaries. We want to be cognizant of that and respectful of the patient's defenses for getting too close to the therapist. Yet if we fail to raise these dynamics with the patient, we risk the therapy languishing. This dynamic, while common with those suffering from BPD, is even more prominent in those with strong narcissistic concerns.

The patient either says everybody else has a problem (which may mean that they do not need to be in therapy, and others should be), or there is something inside them that they may be concerned about and would like to work on. The other issue is that these interactions are sometimes subtle, particularly in patients with identity disturbance, as in the case of Leon. Sometimes, the therapist can blink for a second and could miss it.

"My Father Is Rotten": Fostering a More Integrated Perception of the Other

The second choice point focuses on addressing in-session identity diffusion and how the therapist can foster a more coherent representation of the patient's father. The specific choice point is a situation that begins with a phone call from Leon's wife. She described her husband as emotionally dysregulated and was concerned about his suicidality because he made some thinly veiled threats. Concerned, the therapist called Leon, which the therapist would not normally do. Leon was furious with his father. He ranted about how terrible he is. In his anger, he evoked many strong derogatory phrases about his father, seeing him as rotten to the core.

Transference-Focused Perspective: Addressing Contradictions Without Triggering Vulnerability

From a TFP perspective, we would conceptualize Leon's dysregulated state as stemming from his identity diffusion—the lack of a realistic, consistent, and integrated sense of self and other. From a TFP perspective, it is hypothesized that because of identity disturbance, he cannot represent his experience of himself, his father, and their relationship in a coherent and integrated manner. Given this conceptualization, the question is how do you intervene to help the person become more aware of the disparate aspects of their experience in an effort to become more integrated? We see it as important to gently bring into Leon's awareness the disparate aspects of his experience. Leon vacillated between the disparate parts or representations, often very quickly, as part of identity disturbance. The vacillations between the various representations can happen quickly. One moment Leon said one thing and, at the next, another thing in contrast to what he just said. These vacillations are like watching a ball go back and forth in a ping-pong match and can leave the therapist tired and confused. The patients can feel confused. Other times, either both or one of the people in the dyad can side with one part of the representation and not be aware of the other side. For instance, Leon often talked about his father in an idealized manner. However, when frustrated by him, he would quickly swing into a derogating rant. During either of these states, Leon often did not recognize or recall feeling the other way. So how do you gently bring in the disparate experience in a way that is palatable or at least tolerable to the patient? Often, the material needs to be titrated so it does not leave the patient feeling flooded and overwhelmed or more confused. The therapist may be in a dilemma here because if they do not say anything and let the patient rant, the therapist, in some ways, would reinforce and be taken as endorsing the patient's defensive perspective.

From a TFP perspective, one could see the anger as a defense against the longing: Leon may be longing for his father to be a loving dad with whom he could feel close and intimate. In a metaphor for this impossible relationship, he may feel like Charlie Brown with Lucy and the football in the *Peanuts* comic strip and cartoons: Every time Charlie Brown goes to kick the football, Lucy pulls it away, and he falls flat on his back. Likewise, when Leon seeks emotional support from his father, his father pulls away from him and criticizes him. Leon's anger could be a defense against his sadness about his father and being disappointing to him.

How do you walk that tightrope of bringing into awareness the opposing representations of himself without leaving Leon feeling more vulnerable or exposed? When talking about feelings of vulnerability or longing with patients with narcissistic features, it may be activating to them because it makes them feel so vulnerable. It could be too much for them, flooding and stressing them. It may be like walking across an icy pond—the therapist has to walk across it carefully and quickly because they might break through.

From a TFP perspective, the therapist listens carefully and tracks the narrative of the patient. Issues related to identity disturbance can arise quickly and can be subtle and fleeting. Because such identity issues expressed in the narrative are often difficult to recognize, the therapist has to be attentive and vigilant. It helps if the therapist is integrated and can thus act as an observing ego or therapy historian. The therapist integration allows them to track inconsistencies and vacillations in the patient's narrative that can be raised with the patient and reflected on.

Dialectical Behavior Perspective: Calibrating Interventions Via Patient Vulnerability

To initiate the therapeutic process with Leon, it is crucial to address his distorted perceptions while simultaneously assisting him in regulating his behaviors and emotions. Leon's impulsive and judgmental behaviors, particularly toward his father, likely serve as a means of escaping from unbearable underlying negative emotions, such as hurt, shame, sadness, or loss. Therefore, it is essential to disrupt Leon's avoidance and evasion of these emotions, which may involve helping him interrupt his anger outbursts and judgmental thoughts. The overarching goal is to gradually help Leon develop the capacity to acknowledge, tolerate, and transform the aversive emotions that underlie his symptoms. However, it is of utmost importance for the therapist to navigate this situation in a manner that preserves Leon's sense of safety within the therapeutic relationship because there is a risk of him perceiving the therapist as invalidating.

When confronted with a chaotic and dysregulated patient like Leon, several strategies can prove beneficial, including validation, cognitive modification, motivational techniques, skills training, and a balanced approach that integrates acceptance and change-oriented strategies. The therapist's choice of intervention will be guided, in part, by the patient's vulnerability in each moment. If Leon is exhibiting extreme anger, intense judgment, and disconnection from his underlying painful emotions, the therapist may need to prioritize addressing his defensive behaviors and current emotional expressions. In such cases, the therapist can provide validation by acknowledging the difficulty of resisting the urge to confront his father, stating something like, "It's incredibly challenging not to want to scream at your father." According to the patient's level of vulnerability, the therapist can determine whether additional validation is necessary or if it is possible to guide Leon toward greater awareness of the underlying emotional pain triggered by the situation with his father. If Leon remains highly vulnerable and distanced from his unexpressed painful emotions, the therapist may need to employ acceptance-based techniques, such as further validation and support, expressing understanding with a statement like, "I can see how difficult it is for you to do anything other than judge your father." Throughout the therapeutic process, the therapist must carefully monitor whether the patient perceives any threatening aspects in their interaction and adjust their approach accordingly.

Emotion-Focused Perspective: Shifting From Maladaptive to Adaptive Anger

At this juncture in the psychotherapy, it may be important to highlight the emotional experiences that may be explicating the identity disturbances. This can be done using understanding and interventions from emotion-focused therapy (EFT). From an EFT perspective, differentiating between different types of anger (primary, secondary, or more instrumental) may be necessary. As such, it may be hard for Leon to experience and focus on his more vulnerable emotions (i.e., hurt or sadness), even though this may be the underlying primary experience. Leon may just not be there; he may not be ready or familiar with these emotions. While it seems the identity problems may partially be driven by the hurt he feels by being left alone by his father, he now feels he may be entitled to more or that his father should be with him more often and spend more time with him (given this subjectively felt hurt).

In terms of intervention, a therapeutic focus on Leon's identity-consistent anger would make sense. In EFT terms, this would involve moving from secondary (rejecting) anger to more primary and healthy (assertive) anger; the latter aims to consolidate the boundaries of one's identity and express the underlying need. Working first with the secondary emotions, being empathic and assessing and understanding the function of the secondary anger, Leon learned over his social learning history that to express rejecting anger earns him something: In his development, that expressed anger helped him at some point. Receiving therapist empathy may help tone down the anger a little bit; Leon may still be angry but a little bit less intensely. Then the therapist may say, "It sounds like you're very angry, and I wonder what makes you so angry in this situation." Rather than exploring the hurt right away, the therapist tries to help access the healthier parts of the anger, those that the patient is aware of what makes him angry, and he can stand up for himself and his identity. Instead of accessing the shame or anxiety components, the therapist may foster identity-consistent assertive anger.

SUMMARY STATEMENT: HOW TO MOVE TOWARD AN INTEGRATED SENSE OF SELF

A diffuse and vacillating identity is one of the defining features of personality pathology. Positive progress in psychotherapy for personality disorders is expected to involve a progressive strengthening of identity. Few studies have examined whether change in identity disturbance is a mechanism of change in psychotherapy for personality disorders. Identity is highly interrelated with behavioral impulsivity, emotional dysregulation, and reflective functioning. Identity is not a unitary construct, which makes it difficult to operationalize in a precise manner. In addition, identity overlaps with other functional domains (e.g., impulsivity and emotion dysregulation).

Our discussion of the case of Leon highlights that identity is at the crossroads of integrating information across other functional domains, including problematic emotions, behavior, and interpersonal relationships. It is valuable to consider how to integrate across domains for the best intervention. In Leon's case, the identified choice points suggest two pathways to facilitate change in identity coherence—one focused on the coherent sense of self and one on a coherent perception of the other.

In the first choice point, Leon presents disparate experiences of himself that are out of his awareness. We propose moving in with gentle validation, followed by questioning the patient's momentary experience of himself and the therapist's awareness (and capacity to tolerate in the here and now) that the patient's nonawareness may also be related to the current therapeutic relationship. In the moment, directly addressing the patient's in-session experience and his motivation to change and seeking to understand the meaning of the opposing representations is useful. Independent of the patient's reactions, it may be fruitful for the therapist to recognize the patient's motivation to attain clarity on their attributes, feelings, and desires with self and others. The therapist may need to hold the patient's opposite self-identity until it can be owned by the patient. Patience and emotional maturity are needed to apply these strategies in therapy.

In the second choice point, Leon expresses a harsh and undifferentiated image of his father, and here, several strategies could be employed. The expressed anger may be validated by the therapist. Given the patient's vulnerability, an analogy, such as the one with Charlie Brown and Lucy with the football, could be used to keep things light and accessible to the patient. It is important for the therapist to monitor the patient's emotional vulnerability closely. It is ultimately critical to help Leon attend to and acknowledge underlying avoided emotions, such as feelings of loss and pain. For example, in addition to focusing on Leon's feelings of rejection associated with his anger, the therapist could focus on Leon's primary negative emotions and elements of his assertive anger, which, if mobilized, may help Leon address his needs effectively.

Therapeutic strategies such as the ones described previously, which are used to strengthen a patient's self-identity, need to be studied in greater detail. To date, no studies have directly explored the time-dependent steps of progression from identity confusion to identity coherence. Specific questions to be addressed by future research include: How much therapist validation is necessary when working with identity problems? How effective are confrontational strategies at an early stage of therapy? Is increasing awareness of the initial opposition necessary for the patient to move toward an integrated sense of self? How is the integrated sense of self influenced by the patient's attachment style and other therapist-related factors (i.e., patience and capacity to tolerate frustration and confusion)? These and other questions may be addressed in the future to elucidate the consolidation of identity as a mechanism of change in psychotherapy for personality disorders.

7 MOVING FROM IMPULSIVE BEHAVIOR TO SELF-REFLECTION

Impulsive behavior is a noted symptom of several personality disorders and a core aspect of borderline personality disorder (BPD). Broadly defined, *impulsivity* is a rapid response to internal or external cues without regard for negative consequences associated with action. Poor impulse control can lead to problems in functioning and is, therefore, an important issue to address in psychological treatment. Treating impulsive patients is often challenging for therapists because it can involve high-stakes situations.

This chapter addresses the challenges of treating individuals exhibiting impulsive behavior. There is an extensive body of research on impulsivity from literature in biological psychiatry, personality, and behavior, yet few studies have directly examined changes in various facets of impulsivity as a mechanism of change in psychological treatments of personality disorders. This chapter begins by briefly highlighting the findings from the empirical literature related to mechanisms of change in therapy for personality disorders relevant to impulse control. Next, a case of an 18-year-old adult, Arun, with severe impulsivity, is presented, followed by a discussion of the case

https://doi.org/10.1037/0000388-008
Understanding Mechanisms of Change in Psychotherapies for Personality Disorders, by U. Kramer, K. N. Levy, and S. McMain

formulation from three psychotherapeutic perspectives.[1] The chapter closes with three specific clinical choice points based on discussions between the authors.

EMPIRICAL SUPPORT FOR CHANGES IN FACETS OF IMPULSIVITY AS MECHANISMS OF CHANGE

Reducing behavioral impulsivity and improving the ability to modulate impulsive behavior are favorable outcomes of treatment for personality disorders. Several randomized controlled trials of psychotherapies for personality disorders have assessed changes in impulsive behavior as an outcome of treatment (e.g., Clarkin, Levy, et al., 2007; McMain et al., 2009). Self-harm and suicidal behavior in BPD have received the most attention from researchers; however, other manifestations of impulsivity, including global measures of impulsivity, anger, and substance use have also been investigated. Studies have demonstrated that reduction in impulsive behaviors is associated with improvements on other outcomes (e.g., McMain et al., 2009).

There is some evidence that treatment response may be influenced by baseline levels of impulsivity in borderline individuals. A study by Traynor et al. (2021) found that pretreatment performance-based level of impulsivity, assessed by the Conners' Continuous Performance Test (3rd ed., Conners et al., 2003), was associated with self-harm outcomes in patients diagnosed with BPD. Patients with high pretreatment levels of impulsivity responded better to 6 months of dialectical behavior therapy (DBT) than 12 months of DBT. Patients with lower pretreatment levels of impulsivity responded better to 12 months of DBT than to 6 months of DBT. These findings provide preliminary evidence to suggest that pretreatment neurocognitive performance-based measures of impulsivity may be useful in predicting response to treatment. Thus, patients could be assigned to different treatment doses according to their baseline level of impulsivity.

Research into changes in impulse control as a mechanism of change in psychotherapy for personality disorders is in its infancy. A few studies have examined facets of impulsivity, such as mindfulness and areas of the brain related to executive control. For example, some studies have indirectly examined impulsivity by assessing changes in mindfulness—an attention control strategy that involves focusing one's attention on the present moment while acknowledging and accepting one's experience (e.g., Zeifman et al., 2020). Improvements in

---

[1]The case of Arun has been modified to disguise the patient's identity and protect their confidentiality.

mindfulness are theoretically linked to improvements in impulse control and, consequently, recovery. In addition, studies have examined whether improvements in mindfulness play a role in therapy outcomes in DBT for BPD. For instance, gains in mindfulness have been shown to be associated with reduced health care use and improved emotional well-being in BPD (O'Toole et al., 2012). Other research has indicated that improvements in specific facets of mindfulness—namely nonjudgment—mediate DBT outcomes for patients with BPD. Krantz et al. (2018) found that mindfulness without judgment mediated the effects of 20 weeks of DBT skills training on self-harm outcomes. Using the same sample, Zeifman et al. (2020) also found that improvements in mindfulness—particularly mindfulness without judgment—mediated improvements in general psychopathology measures after 20 weeks of DBT skills training for BPD.

Other research involving neuroimaging techniques has examined changes in the brain related to impulsivity and treatment outcomes in individuals with personality disorders. Research provided preliminary support indicating that changes in the neurocircuitry of the brain related to impulsivity are linked to favorable psychotherapy outcomes in the treatment of personality disorders. Using functional magnetic resonance imaging, Schmitt et al. (2016) found that 12 weeks of DBT for BPD resulted in increased frontal-limbic connectivity and increased grey matter. Twelve weeks of DBT for BPD has also been linked to increases in grey matter in the anterior cingulate cortex (Mancke et al., 2018). Using the go–no-go paradigm, Perez et al. (2016) showed consistent effects in favor of enhanced frontolimbic connectivity after 1-year-long transference-focused psychotherapy (TFP) for 10 patients with BPD.

In sum, some evidence has demonstrated that improvements in mindfulness, a construct relevant to impulsivity, as well as brain activity (e.g., frontolimbic connectivity), may explain the effects of psychotherapy for personality disorders. In the next section, we consider how impulsive symptoms manifest in an individual and how to guide treatment interventions to reduce these problems and open a path to improved self-reflection.

THE CASE OF ARUN

Arun is an 18-year-old single male diagnosed with multiple psychiatric disorders, including BPD, antisocial personality disorder (ASPD), attention-deficit/hyperactivity disorder, and polysubstance use disorders. He has a lengthy history of self-harm behaviors, involving mostly low lethality cutting and overdoses, in addition to three suicide attempts. He has abused alcohol, marijuana, cocaine, and occasionally amphetamines for a long time. Arun lives alone in a rented room and is supported by disability benefits.

Arun was referred to a specialist BPD outpatient treatment program after being discharged from an adolescent residential program because of his stalking and harassment of female patients. He agreed to engage in an out-patient DBT program that included attending weekly individual therapy, skills training, and out-of-session phone coaching to manage crises. Initially, skills training was delivered to him on an individual rather than group basis because of concerns about his risk of stalking and harassing other group patients.

At the start of the treatment, his behavior was characterized by frequent crises, such as suicide threats; emergency room visits; substance abuse, including an overdose; frequent self-harm behavior; sexual promiscuity; verbal and physical altercations with others; and excessive texting and stalking of people. His anger outbursts were typically intense and characterized by threats to kill himself or others, occasionally leading to physical altercations and property destruction. Arun's suicidality and anger outbursts were usually triggered by perceived rejection by others.

Arun is the eldest child in an intact family with four siblings. He has three younger sisters. His parents immigrated to North America with their four children after fleeing a violent and politically oppressive regime in South Asia. His family endured numerous tragedies and traumatic experiences. According to Arun's accounts, his parents exhibited posttraumatic stress symptoms. Arun recounted repeated emotionally invalidating and physically traumatic experiences during his childhood. His parents often erupted unpredictably into fits of rage with one another and with Arun and his siblings. His father drank heavily and frequently became violent with Arun when drunk, leading Arun to flee the home to escape the abuse. Child welfare authorities were involved with the family when Arun was 10 and, at this time, he was removed from the home for 1 year. This contributed to a sense of neglect and abandonment, as well as a belief that there was something wrong or bad with him. He often felt scared and angry about how he was treated and was concerned about protecting himself.

Arun presented to his first therapy session on time. His mood was labile: he appeared anxious and displayed motor tics, such as ear pulling and throat clearing. He talked rapidly and excessively. The therapist found it difficult to talk without interrupting him. Arun appeared anxious and mistrustful, though he was friendly and smiled often. It was difficult for Arun to focus on any topic for long, and the conversation frequently shifted between topics. In a jubilant manner, he expressed his excitement about his diagnosis of BPD because he thought it characterized him well. He believed he had been misdiagnosed all his life. In response to questions about what he wanted help with in therapy, he expressed a desire to have stable relationships with people, especially women. He spoke unabashedly about his problems with repeatedly texting people and stalking them. He excitedly described in detail how he had threatened people, punched walls in anger, and frequently fantasized about harming people. When he spoke about women and how they frequently rebuffed his advances, he became visibly angry. He described himself as an "emotional person" and someone who struggled to control his behavior. He seemed eager to make a positive impression on the therapist and spoke with bravado about his aggressive behavior.

CASE FORMULATION: UNDERSTANDING THE ROOTS OF IMPULSIVE BEHAVIORS

In this section, we turn to the case formulation from different perspectives in an attempt to explain the variety of impulsive behaviors displayed by Arun.

Dialectical Behavior Formulation: The Role of Repeated Trauma and Invalidation

Arun's symptoms can be understood within the framework of DBT as stemming from pervasive deficits in emotion regulation. Undoubtedly, environmental factors have played a significant role in contributing to Arun's difficulties in regulating his emotions. He shared a history of repeated childhood traumatic experiences, including physical abuse that led to his removal from his home by child welfare authorities. In addition, he described numerous instances of emotional invalidation, where his reactions were trivialized and ignored, and he was often blamed for his experiences.

The development of an individual's emotion regulation capacities is influenced by a complex interplay between biological and environmental factors. In Arun's case, both his parents have mental health and addiction issues. While genetic factors may contribute to the development of emotion regulation deficits, the impact of invalidating environmental experiences is prominent in Arun's history.

Arun's repeated traumatic and invalidating experiences are likely major factors contributing to his difficulties in emotion regulation. He may have failed to learn how to acknowledge and accept painful emotions and lacked opportunities to regulate his emotional experiences and communicate his emotional needs effectively. Faced with physical abuse, Arun likely experienced feelings of terror, helplessness, and powerlessness that were overwhelming for a child to endure. The absence of a compassionate and soothing caregiver to support him during these distressing emotions hindered his ability to learn self-soothing techniques. In addition, asserting his emotional needs may have been perceived as risky, given his parents' unpredictable anger outbursts in response to such expressions. Consequently, aversive emotions associated with traumatic experiences, such as shame, powerlessness, and helplessness, were likely avoided and eventually intensified over time.

Feelings of aloneness and mistrust of others are common consequences of childhood maltreatment. Arun may have developed maladaptive coping strategies, such as impulsive behavior, to escape the underlying painful emotional experiences. For example, his explosive anger and homicidal thoughts may serve as a way to flee from overwhelming feelings of powerlessness and aloneness and a deep-seated belief in his inherent flaws. Arun's interactions with others are likely to trigger underlying painful emotions, such as shame and disappointment. He may anticipate rejection from others and perceive threat cues even when no real threat is present. Consequently, when these aversive emotions are activated, Arun typically seeks to escape through impulsive behaviors, including anger outbursts, sexual promiscuity, and substance abuse.

The overarching goal of therapy for Arun is to assist him in learning effective emotion regulation strategies and increase his capacity to tolerate the chronically avoided emotional experiences that underlie his symptoms.

Transference-Focused Formulation: Understanding the Scope of the Patient's Problems and Self-Awareness

The case formulation or conceptualization is not only important for the therapist as a guide but is also important for establishing an explicit treatment framework with the patient. This requires knowledge of the scope of the patient's difficulties, so the therapist can share an initial understanding or conceptualization of the difficulties and can speculate on the underlying reasons for them. This framework or case conceptualization serves the discussion between the patient's and therapist's roles and responsibilities over the course of the treatment. This requires engaging in a collaborative and nonjudgmental manner. From a TFP perspective, Arun's impulsive behavior is seen as a defensive process and avoidance of uncomfortable emotional states. We would see the impulsive behaviors as a result of being activated by feelings or beliefs, such as feeling unattended to or embarrassed or that others may not have their best interest at heart. These thoughts and feelings can be activated on the basis of an accurate understanding of the interaction with another, or they can represent misinterpretations of others' intentions or behaviors.

Regardless, the patient lacks internal psychological structures to contextualize the experience as someone without a personality disorder might. From a mentalization-based therapy perspective, psychological capacity is seen as the capacity to mentalize one's own and others' minds and to make accurate attributions about them. Thus, the therapist may see Arun's feelings of neglect and shame as resulting from someone not seeing him the way he wants to be seen, which is representative of his challenges. There is also an ongoing process that leads him to want to shed and avoid those feelings. The patient acts impulsively as a way of getting past those feelings.

The therapist would point out to the patient their reactions to social and environmental stimuli and assess whether the patient is aware of how they are reacting to get a sense of their insight into and awareness of their behavior. For example, when a patient tells a therapist about something terrible that has happened in their life with a big smile on their face, the therapist may point out, "I'm not sure if this is meaningful or if you're aware of it, but as you were telling me about this, you have a smile on your face. I wonder if we could think about what might be going on or what that might be about." The therapist assesses whether the patient realizes they are smiling when discussing trauma to gauge their insight into their behavior. Some people have nuanced understandings of their behavior, and while some insights are believable, others are contrived. A response that may emerge is, "I'm smiling because it's so tragic." In this instance, the patient's statement does not provide a nuanced understanding and may be meant to cut off the process rather than deepen it. Regardless of the patient's conscious motivations, the patient's statement is canned, almost cliché, and does not provide much information to the therapist. The therapist can use the principle articulated earlier by focusing on the patient's response to help them develop greater awareness of their experience. The therapist continues to engage the patient to develop a deeper case formulation.

The therapist emphasizes the importance of collaboration in the therapeutic process. If the patient does experience the therapist as imposing something on them or controlling them, in the therapist's mind, it is something that can be assessed. In psychoanalytic terms, the therapist often interprets that, but it essentially entails assessing whether the therapist was being controlling. If the therapist acts in a way that could be interpreted as imposing or controlling, they can no longer judge whether the patient's reactions are reasonable. This is one of the reasons the therapist tries to keep their perspective nonjudgmental and neutral. The therapist wants to be able to judge whether the patient's reaction accurately reflects what has happened in the therapy room or is a distortion that might be meaningful for thinking about the therapy. The consequences extend even outside of therapy because if the patient distorts the therapist's behaviors, they might distort experiences with other people in their lives in that way, too.

Arun's case was discussed diagnostically, and it was determined that he meets the criteria for BPD and ASPD. Although he did not meet the full criteria, he also displayed characteristics consistent with narcissism. For example, he had a strong need to be admired, to be the focus of attention, and he showed an inability to tolerate even the slightest indications that somebody might not be holding him to the ideal that he desired to be held to. When working with those high in narcissism or with prominent narcissistic concerns, it is important for the therapist to be careful about the wording of interventions to avoid offending the patient. Those high in narcissism tend to be much more sensitive and brittle in therapy. These dynamics aid the therapist in the case formulation and help guide interventions. When narcissistic concerns are present, the therapist must ensure that what they say cannot be easily misinterpreted. If the therapist uses language carefully, any misinterpretation by the patient can be used in the case formulation.

Plan Analysis Formulation: Understanding the Motives Behind the Impulsive Behavior

Arun's clinical presentation is particularly challenging, and a careful case formulation could help to understand the possible motivational underpinnings of his contrasting behaviors. It appears that, clinically, Arun acts on the spur of the moment, yet he has an overall self-presentation of being someone cool, likable, and in charge. Both threads may be explained by underlying purposes determined by plan analysis (Caspar, 2019). If Arun's impulsivity has an instrumental component, one could speculate that he would make rash decisions to feel in control and modulate his emotions (while at the same time acting out has uncontrollable effects on the interaction). Plans such as "control your emotions," "make sure the other person sees you in your impulsive behavior," and "act as if you are in control" are likely to be found in Arun's plan analytic case conceptualization.

Given this complexity and the potentially harmful consequences of Arun's impulsive behaviors, it would be difficult but feasible to intervene using the motive-oriented therapeutic relationship (MOTR). The therapist should focus on the level of the motives without reinforcing the problematic coping plans shown by this patient. For example, if the plan "impress the other" (with some "cool" attitude) is activated in the interaction, such as in the first session described in the case presentation, the therapist would conceptualize this plan as serving a higher plan, such as "make sure the other remains oriented toward me," or "make sure the other person takes care of me." The latter two may be acceptable motives, potentially explaining some of the motivational underpinnings of the more problematic means to these ends. Therapists who are being complementary on the level of the motives will potentially remove the motivational basis of the problematic means, making them superfluous. The MOTR therapist may say, "Wow, there are so many dangerous behaviors you engage in, Arun, and it seems to me that it is important to you to come in to see me. I notice you are on time today. So, I am glad you are here today, so we can, if you agree, figure out together how I can help you best with some of these behaviors. Which behavior you engage in should we start with?" This intervention would be highly oriented toward Arun's likely activated motives, yet at the same time, signify the context of help (and its limits) and directly orient to the need to define a clear mission (or goal) of this therapy.

Talking about different impulsive behaviors, Arun described various problematic states, some of which he is experiencing in the moment. Addressing these behaviors is important, but the therapist is also aware that there are likely two levels to consider: the primary focus and the secondary. The main productive focus may be related to the core underlying problem, which is currently unclear. At this point, what is evident is that the therapist and patient are in an interpersonal dynamic, and the presenting problems (e.g., impulsivity, rash decisions, passivity) may not be the main issue. While his impulsive behavior is significant and needs to be targeted quickly, it is likely secondary to a deeper core emotional issue. The core issue is likely a chronic sense of being left out, not belonging, or not having a place in his family. Leaving his family was likely devastating for Arun; he reported that although the family was intact, he had never experienced a sense of togetherness. More information is needed to determine what is underlying this.

Thus, the case formulation of this patient needs to address these two levels: the core problem underlying the behaviors and the expressed symptoms. Clinicians with less experience may think they need to shift immediate focus to the deeper core issues underlying the symptoms, but while they are important and central, such a therapeutic move may be premature at this juncture.

Toward a Common Formulation

Despite some differences in our conceptual emphases, the three formulations shared important features. First, each approach conceptualized Arun's impulsive behavior as a maladaptive symptom that protects him from underlying vulnerable emotions. Arun's impulsive aggressive behavior can be viewed as a defensive yet adaptive response that protects him from emotion vulnerabilities and a perceived defective sense of self. Accordingly, a treatment implication of this shared perspective is the importance of focusing on multiple levels, including Arun's overt symptoms and the underlying vulnerabilities.

Second, focusing on the etiology of Arun's impulsive behavior, each method highlighted the contributing role of his pervasive, traumatically invalidating childhood experiences. For example, each author identified the presence of intense negative emotions, a poor sense of self, and deficits in emotion regulation capacities that developed as consequences of interpersonally invalidating experiences.

As noted, each formulation differed in some important ways. In contrast to the other approaches, the plan analytic perspective is based on an analysis of Arun's relational motives and places a greater emphasis on the interpersonal function of his behavior, theorizing that Arun's aggressive behavior may be motivated by a need for interpersonal connection with others. The transference-focused perspective concentrates on Arun's perceptions in response to social and environmental stimuli. In keeping with the DBT emphasis on emotions, the dialectical behavior perspective focused on the role of emotions, particularly the role of deficits in emotional regulation underlying impulsive behaviors.

CHOICE POINTS AND OPPORTUNITIES FOR CHANGE

In this section, we discuss how we would intervene at three choice points based on our formulation and any related empirical evidence concerning the treatment of impulsivity. The first concerns the therapist knowing what to do if the patient abruptly changes topics in the session. The second relates to in-session intense agitation related to a distressing narrative. The third concerns a choice point that arose when the therapist directly asked for advice. Table 7.1 synthesizes generic and approach-specific strategies that therapists might use, as well as relevant patient processes, in the three choice points presented in this chapter.

"Let's Go to the Bar!": Addressing an Impulsive Shift of Topic

Arun presented 35 minutes late to his second session. Upon entering the therapy room, he sat down and texted for several minutes before looking up from his cell phone. His mood was upbeat, and he delightfully described how he rode his bicycle to the session and intentionally swerved in front of a truck driver just to "piss him off." He explained that he reacted justifiably in this manner because the truck driver had tried to cut him off. The therapist struggled to keep a focus in session because Arun jumped back and forth in his narration. At one point, Arun launched into a long diatribe about a young woman he tried to "hook" up with. He expressed irritation with her after he

TABLE 7.1. How to Foster a Path to Self-Reflectivity

Generic therapist interventions	Specific therapist interventions	Patient processes
Choice point: Addressing impulsive shifts of topic		
• Establish the treatment frame. • Validate the valid. • Target lack of direction. • Observe counter-transference.	• Develop goals. • Express curiosity. • Express empathy and interest. • Target underlying motives. • Focus on the therapist's feelings.	• Reduce emotion arousal; increase attention. • Learn to be transparent about behavior. • Self-validate. • Be aware of self-direction. • Be aware of in-session feelings.
Choice point: Addressing in-session agitation		
• Monitor negative reactions or counter-transference. • Structure the session. • Use dialectical strategies. • Intervene on the relationship level.	• Slow down, express with calm and measured voice, engage in self-disclosure. • Set limits if needed. • Balance challenge and validation. • Focus on underlying motives.	• Reduce emotional arousal. • Slow down. • Increase awareness while feeling accepted. • Increase awareness of behaviors in relation to others.
Choice point: Addressing request for advice		
• Promote awareness in the patient. • Use dialectical strategies. • Highlight underlying motives and emotional needs.	• Offer a reflection of experience. • Balance a focus on validation and change. • Use the motive-oriented therapeutic relationship.	• Increase awareness of thoughts, emotions, and behaviors. • Increase attention and awareness of in-session requests. • Increase awareness of needs.

invited her out on a date, and she responded flatly and unenthusiastically with the word "okay." He concluded that she was not interested in him. Midway through this story, he abruptly shifted topics and described a drug-induced, angry escapade with friends:

> And then I called up some friends and said, "My parents are driving me nuts; let's go to the bar." It was supposed to be an hour thing, and it turned into bar hopping from bar to bar, and I had quite a few shots. My friend offered me a few lines of amphetamine and everything, and then, all of a sudden, I'm on this group chat with a bunch of other people with mental health issues, and I said some pretty messed up stuff. Then one of my other friends, my ex, who has BPD, said, "Arun, are you okay? You're saying things that are a little offensive and a little bit . . . off." She didn't like it when I said, "Hey, call my

new number." It wasn't actually my number; it was this girl that I wanted to mess with. And then the girl with BPD said, "Dude, that's horrible. Why the fuck would you want to do that?" Then she started messing with me, saying, "Hey, if you do that again, we'll have to get you arrested because you can't get away with that stuff."

Plan Analysis Perspective: Structuring the Patient's Narrative

In this excerpt, it seems important for the therapist to be aware that it seems like an effort for Arun to come back to the therapy session, given the instability in his clinical presentation and the major task of this session (and the following ones) is relationship building between the therapist and patient. It would be premature, at Session 2, in this case, to move into therapeutic work on the specific contents of therapy, but the patient needs to see and feel that this is a potentially helpful space for him. Given this initial goal, the therapist may intervene by slowing the patient down. Arun's self-interruption of the first topic (i.e., the hook-up with a girl, which is consistent with his upbeat and more positive self-presentation, with a likely activated plan of "presenting as cool to the therapist"), moving abruptly to discussing the situation about drug use and the expressed anger with friends, may be problematic. The therapist may want to intervene right after this self-interruption and say, "I am lost, and I want to get this right. I am interested in what you say about the drug use at the bar, but I want to stick with your story about this girl—were you interested in this girl or not?" This may help to focus on the unfinished narrative and finish it before moving to the second one.

Then, after offering this structure, the second narrative is potentially more problematic than the first one and highly relevant to the functional domain of impulsivity because it involves the patient's rash behavior. A motive-oriented therapist may need to say at some point, "It sounds like you were in several quite dangerous situations while at this bar. I assume you were doing your best in these situations, but they can be tricky for you and others. Can you say more about how you made the decision to take a few lines of amphetamines at this one bar the other night?"

While the therapist focuses on the underlying motive that would likely be high in Arun's plan structure (i.e., complementarity to a plan such as "present as somebody good," "make sure to get the therapist's attention," "present as cool," "avoid being judged by others"), given the high risks involved in Arun's behavior, it may be sound also to explore some of the difficult ("tricky") situations and their (potentially dangerous) consequences on Arun's health. The latter therapeutic move will become key in developing a stringent and stable therapy focus (i.e., the mission to mutually agree on tasks and goals of this therapy). A MOTR therapist would be aware that Arun needs his relationship with his therapist to be stronger at this point than it currently is, and any move toward defining a problematic behavior too quickly may be met by even more impulsive reactions by the patient in the session.

Transference-Focused Perspective: Encourage Self-Reflection
The patient was telling a story about what happened on his way to the session when he quickly shifted to talking about his mother. The TFP therapist would pay attention to the "domino effect," the interpersonal dynamics between the patient and the therapist, and the affective component in the room. Initially, the therapist would perceive the patient as upbeat and focused on impressing them. Another interpretation of this scenario is that the patient is attempting to avoid difficult and upsetting topics. The patient was angry, yet he presented as though he was not angry and was in control. It would be important to slow down the process to help the patient sit more with what he was experiencing, even if it would just be incremental. The goal would be to help the patient reflect more on what was happening.

One of the things we pay attention to from the TFP perspective is how what Arun expressed is representational. This was apparent when he talked about the women, his mother, or the truck driver who cut him off. We are looking for how he sees himself in relation to others and how he sees others. In some ways, we can note that there are similar patterns and that he vacillates between two different perspectives. The therapist seeks to understand the dynamic of not being able to tolerate uncomfortable feelings.

A transference-focused therapist would agree with the approaches of a plan analyst and dialectical behavior therapist. However, if this is the issue, it is important to know what you are doing as a therapist and ensure there is a purpose to what is being done versus what is not, for lack of a better way.

As for countertransference or emotional reaction to the patient, from a TFP approach, it would be essential to clarify what happened, in part because he could have killed somebody. The other issue is that when Arun talks about what happened, the therapist can hear the nuances of disparate aspects of his experience that we find useful. In some ways, the devil is in the details there. Patients use certain constituents as part of a kind of transference or reaction when they become cavalier about the therapy. The same intervention could look similar or different, depending on how the therapist uses it. Therapists who treat those with BPD are often afraid that the biggest countertransferential reaction they will have is to become angry with patients. However, the most common enactment in therapy with patients with BPD is therapist passivity. Rather than getting angry with patients, therapists defend against the anger and become passive. The passivity results in the therapist just sitting there, waiting for sessions to end, and not doing the hard work of therapy.

A therapist might pass the time by asking questions like, "Tell me about what happened," not because they want to understand the details or scope of the patient's experience but because they are avoiding conflictual discourse. Likewise, therapists will sometimes ask about childhood relationships with parents or make interpretations about the role of early childhood relationships because it is easy to do and deflects the patient from difficult material in the therapeutic relationship.

Dialectical Behavior Perspective: Modulate the Patient's Emotions

When faced with Arun's communication, it is crucial for the therapist to approach the situation with attentive listening and a genuine desire to understand the patient while assisting Arun in regulating his overwhelming emotions and gaining insight into his behavior.

Arun entered the session with heightened energy and intense emotions, making it essential for the therapist to address the immediate emotional state and facilitate emotion regulation. Arun's rapid and excessive speech can indicate a need for focused attention on his emotional arousal. Validating Arun's experience and conveying understanding become valuable tools in promoting self-regulation.

To begin, the therapist can offer validation by acknowledging Arun's emotions, his difficulty in managing emotions, and the intensity of his arousal. This validation would help Arun feel heard and understood, creating a sense of safety within the therapeutic relationship. For instance, if the patient exclaims, "My parents are driving me nuts," the therapist can respond with empathy, saying, "It sounds like something about your interactions with your parents might have been hurtful or disappointing."

Furthermore, the therapist can pay close attention to the content of the patient's narrative, actively listening for cues that reveal underlying avoided emotions. By doing so, the therapist can guide the patient's awareness of these emotions, facilitating their exploration and expression. For instance, if the patient describes a frustrating situation, the therapist can gently highlight the potential hurt or disappointment that may be present, helping the patient recognize and engage with their emotional experiences.

In addition to validation and exploration, the therapist can support the patient in increasing their emotional awareness by helping them observe and describe their emotions. By encouraging the patient to identify and label their emotions in the moment, the therapist helps promote emotion regulation and self-understanding.

Attending to the patient's heightened emotional arousal is crucial because it can impede their ability to process information and actively participate in therapy. Collaboratively engaging the patient in observing and modulating their intense emotions is helpful. The therapist can gently suggest slowing down and taking deep breaths, allowing the patient to regain control and better understand the situation. Using a collaborative tone rather than being directive or controlling is important in preventing defensiveness and heightening emotional arousal.

Another effective approach in such situations is to employ a dialectical response that encourages self-reflection. By responding unexpectedly and irreverently with a confrontational tone, the therapist can help shift the patient's attention and reduce emotional arousal. For example, the therapist might say, "Are you out of your mind? This sounds like a crazy situation." This approach can be used to disrupt the patient's current track and promote self-reflection.

When working with a highly emotionally dysregulated patient like Arun, it is crucial to be cautious with using directive strategies that may increase their sense of threat. If directive interventions are necessary, they should be embedded in validating communication. For instance, if the patient's voice becomes raised and disruptive, the therapist can acknowledge their frustration while kindly requesting them to speak more softly to ensure others are not disturbed.

Considering this is only the second session with Arun, it is important to establish the focus and frame of therapy. This involves determining the range and severity of Arun's presenting problems. In DBT, treatment targets are prioritized based on their level of risk. Assessing the patient's problems directly and exploring their goals is essential. The therapist should inquire about any undisclosed issues that may be too shameful to discuss, exploring precipitants and consequences of specific behaviors to gain insight into what controls the patient's problems.

Once the scope and nature of Arun's problems are identified, the therapist's task is to establish mutually determined goals for therapy. This requires exploring Arun's motivation to work on these problems because low motivation to change is not uncommon. Strengthening the patient's motivation and commitment to eliminating life-threatening behaviors and increasing engagement in treatment becomes a priority. Strategies such as exploring the pros and cons of change or using the devil's advocate technique (Linehan, 1993) can be employed to enhance motivation. If the patient is unwilling to work on specific goals or tasks, the therapist needs to assess the viability of the treatment without their willingness. Ultimately, it is the patient's life, and the therapist's role is not to impose their goals but to support the patient in achieving their desired outcomes.

"She Says to Me, 'Lazy Fucking Asshole'": Addressing In-Session Agitation Related to a Distressing Narrative

Arun frequently presented to session in an angry mood, usually triggered by perceived criticism from others. At Session 7, he appeared agitated when the therapist met him in the waiting room. He expressed irritation about a bus driver and anger toward the receptionist. While walking down the hallway to the therapist's office, he began loudly complaining about his parents. Arun's diatribe was drawing the attention of others close by. The therapist worked to help contain the conversation and his anger, at least until they were in the privacy of the therapy office. Upon entry to the office, he immediately launched into a detailed account of a fight he just had with his mother.

> [*Talking rapidly*] Well, I just smashed some things, and then she says to me, "Oh, it's your diagnosis; it's an excuse for you to be such a lazy fucking asshole." I'm like, "Oh, my God, you do realize that mental health is genetic, right? You realize that it's genetic, right?" I'm pretty sure that she's got some of the same problems.

Transference-Focused Perspective: Addressing Countertransference and Being Present

The therapist may feel overwhelmed at this juncture of the psychotherapy. A therapist who feels overwhelmed would talk about their experience to target the countertransference or any countertransference enactment. When a therapist feels overwhelmed by the patient, they may feel as if they want to help the patient and then move into a quicker action than might otherwise be indicated. The therapist reacting to what is happening in the room, coloring how they feel they need to respond, is a common occurrence.

The issue of being controlling is central because it can be seen as an enactment that the therapist could easily fall into. This would then lead Arun to feel the way he does with his mother and other women when he perceives that they are in control and he does not have control. There are several ways to approach this, and as in DBT, a transference-focused therapist would help a patient slow down. The therapist would need to ensure they do not present themself as imposing something on the patient, controlling them, or being an authority. This can be subtle and as simple as modeling slowing down or saying, "Hmm, that's interesting," to gently interrupt the patient in their process.

Another optimal approach for the therapist would be to comment about what is happening in the moment—for example, pointing out how much the patient is aware of. The therapist might reflect, "There's a lot of energy here. I'm wondering if you're aware of that, too." This statement is intended to enhance awareness and reflection, which would otherwise be understood as mindfulness from a DBT approach. To draw a patient's awareness to what is happening in the moment, the therapist might say, "I notice as we're talking that you're getting very animated, and clearly, this is important to you. But I'm wondering if you have a sense of that, too." The therapist might also ask the patient if they understand what makes it so important to them.

When a patient becomes forceful with the information they are presenting, a therapist could interpret that the patient thinks no one would believe them otherwise. However, premature interpretation is a common mistake that therapists make. Instead, it would be important to work toward experiencing the patient and encouraging them to experience themselves in the moment. A transference-focused therapist would prioritize slowing down, allowing the patient to reflect, and checking in on the patient's awareness of their experience. Eventually, this would progress to thinking about what a precipitant might be or how the dynamic within the interpersonal process of therapy activates the experience. While Arun talks about his mother and the other women, it is important to recognize that the dynamic is also happening in the moment at some level that the therapist could comment on.

While it is important to avoid an authoritative or expert position as a therapist, it is evident that Arun is being impulsive, and the therapist is not. The two are naturally in different positions. The therapist could try to connect with Arun by stepping up symbolically to meet him and remind him that the therapist is present and listening. A transference-focused therapist would want to interrupt this monologue to say, "Can you just look at me? Can you just see that I'm here?" By starting there, the focus can be narrowed to what is going on inside this patient or between the therapist and patient. The focus should be less on technique and more on being present. It is imperative for a therapist to assert their presence. As necessary, the therapist might even stand in the way of a patient's monologue, interrupt the patient, and remind the patient that there is somebody in the room who is attending to them. This introduces a sense of the other.

Dialectical Behavior Perspective: Regulating Therapist and Patient Emotions

Working with a patient like Arun, whose behavior is impulsive, disruptive, and dangerous, can be a significant challenge for therapists. It is natural to feel fear and become emotionally overwhelmed in the face of such high-risk behavior. However, it is crucial for therapists to regulate their emotions to work with the patient effectively. Acting out of fear and urgency to quickly change the patient's behavior can exacerbate their emotional dysregulation and hinder their engagement in therapy.

Helping impulsive and emotionally dysregulated patients learn to modulate their emotions is an essential aspect of therapy. Simply allowing the patient to vent their anger without direction is not productive. Validation is a valuable strategy that promotes the patient's engagement and self-regulation. It involves actively listening, understanding the core of the problem, and conveying the reasonableness or wisdom in the patient's response. When a patient speaks rapidly, excessively, and loudly, the therapist can validate their present emotional experience, acknowledge the intensity of their frustration, and empathize with their difficulty in controlling their urge to yell. Validation helps reduce emotional arousal, builds a stronger therapeutic bond, and increases the patient's collaboration. Moreover, it facilitates the patient's awareness and acceptance of their experience.

Working with an angry patient requires the therapist to monitor their own emotional reactions to ensure they do not interfere with the treatment process. In this situation, the therapist may feel overwhelmed by Arun's rapid speech and raised voice. They might experience heightened emotional arousal, a sense of pressure, and an urgency to prevent the patient from engaging in dangerous actions. At times, it may feel like watching someone drive a car toward a cliff, leaving the therapist feeling helpless and ineffective. It is essential for the therapist to employ strategies such as mindfulness to counteract these reactions. By monitoring and modulating their own reactions, therapists can prevent themselves from acting impulsively based on fear, allowing for a more effective therapeutic approach.

Self-disclosure can be a helpful tool for therapists to regulate their emotional reactions. For example, the therapist may choose to disclose their feelings by saying, "What you're sharing with me feels incredibly important, and I genuinely want to understand. However, I'm feeling overwhelmed by the intensity of your words, and it's challenging for me to process everything at once. It would be helpful if we could slow down the pace so that I can fully grasp what you're saying." This approach involves the therapist speaking sincerely and directly while also acknowledging their personal limits.

When using self-disclosure, the way the therapist expresses their feelings is crucial. It is important for the therapist to aim at reducing any power differential and perceived sense of threat. Adopting a more one-down stance in the therapeutic relationship can be beneficial. For instance, the therapist might say, "I apologize if I seem a bit slow in processing your words. I want to make sure I understand you fully, so could you please slow down a little to accommodate my pace." This approach helps create a sense of collaboration, decreases the power differential between the therapist and the patient, and helps to foster a safer and more productive therapeutic environment.

In DBT, the therapist aims to strike a balance between validation and promoting behavioral change. In this case, the therapist can help Arun develop more adaptive coping behaviors to regulate his emotional arousal. DBT provides a range of coping skills that can be valuable in such situations. For instance, the therapist could intervene by inviting patients to actively reduce their emotional arousal through deep breathing. An example of this approach might be, "Would you be open to slowing down for a moment? Perhaps we can take a few deep breaths together." This gentle suggestion empowers the patient to engage in a self-regulating practice without feeling pressured or controlled. By incorporating the patient's willingness and participation, the therapist fosters a collaborative atmosphere and encourages the development of adaptive coping strategies.

Plan Analysis Perspective: Focus on Underlying Motives, Not Maladaptive Coping

From a motive-oriented therapeutic approach, the therapist would be interested in the expression of the invalidating comments Arun made to his mother. What is the purpose of Arun storming into the therapy room and expressing the invalidating statements of his mother? A couple of different hypothetical plans come to mind. For example, the patient may want to express this invalidation to evoke sympathy in the therapist, irrespective of the fact that this may or may not be the therapist's reaction. Or it could be explained by a plan such as "present as cool" (to this therapist, to whom the patient may dare say anything, including nasty things about his mother). In addition, it could also be an indirect way of expressing some concern about his own mental health (when he said to his mother that "it is genetic"), which could reflect a plan such as "present as somebody in need of help" or as the motive of "seek help."

A MOTR-informed therapist could take up some of these hypothetically activated plans in their intervention with Arun by focusing on the acceptable underlying motives. For example, the therapist may (by being complementary to the motive of "seek help"), by inserting some paradox, say, "It sounds like you need help with some health issues. You express your need all over, including to your mom and even loudly in the waiting room, right? If you agree, we could have a closer look at how we can help you learn how to express your need for help better. I will be here to support you in this." Explicitly addressing the underlying motives in this way and satisfying some of them while not focusing directly on the more problematic coping plans reflect the lower levels in the plan structure. This approach may help the patient form a new corrective relationship experience while simultaneously focusing on the problematic issue they have brought to therapy. Arun may have never experienced someone who said calmly to him, "I will be here to support you in this," but may have experienced previous therapists either offering complex theories about his functioning or subjectively unhelpful solutions. Arun's behavior in this situation suggests that underlying motive is not to receive a solution nor have new insights right away but to have someone in his context on whom he can rely and who can contain the disruptive and "loud" behaviors.

"What Do You Think?": How to Intervene When Directly Asked for Advice

Arun presented to Session 10 appearing to be in a good mood. He immediately began proudly informing the therapist that he met a woman at a bar the previous night and thinks she is great. She gave him her phone number, but he was not sure how to interpret her behavior. Seeking reassurance, he asked the therapist if this meant that the woman liked him.

> What do you think? Or maybe she's some sick fuck that does this to all the guys. Do you think she's just messing with me? I sort of thought that she was interested in me. Why else would she give me her number? Do you think I should call her and ask her out, or is it too soon? Maybe she thinks I'm stalking her?

Transference-Focused Perspective: Clarify the Patient's Experience

From a TFP or a more broadly dynamic perspective, a therapist could approach the patient in several ways similar to a plan analytic and DBT approach. The therapist would be hesitant to use the word *validation* because people sometimes do not understand the nuance and subtlety of what it means. When used imprecisely, a therapist can risk validating distortions in the patient's experience. Therapists must be skilled in not validating what might be a distortion in a patient's experience; however, this is an easy trap to fall into.

In addition, validation is not always reassuring to patients, partly because they have their own doubts. When a therapist validates something by saying, "Well, it sounds like you had a good reason to feel upset," there may be a part of the patient that feels, "Yeah, that's true. I had a good reason." However, there may be another part of a patient that doubts they had a legitimate reason, or they might be withholding something from you. This would belie them having as good a reason as the therapist might have thought, and it essentially tells them that the therapist does not fully understand their experience.

Clinically, a transference-focused therapist would employ techniques consistent with a general psychodynamic model. The therapist would seek clarification surrounding the patient's experience and not assume an understanding of what the patient means. An example would be in the case of a patient who says, "I'm depressed." Depression can mean feeling depressed, but it can also mean a lot of different things. A therapist might think they know what the patient means when they do not. The therapist must prioritize clarifying the patient's phenomenological experience. When a therapist starts clarifying, there is much more subtlety and nuance to what the patient is expressing and where the disparities arise in their experience. It is those disparities that a therapist attempts to gently bring into the patient's awareness, not just mentally, so that the patient can grapple with them. Again, this must be titrated often to avoid overwhelming the patient by being 20 moves ahead.

Arun strongly desires to be admired, valued, and potentially put on a pedestal. He feels ignored and discarded. It would not be appropriate for a therapist to talk about Arun's vulnerabilities and needs early on in a way that might overwhelm him. This would manifest in session as the patient wanting to be valued by the therapist as well. Arun tells his story in a bravado way and nonchalantly blurts out traumatic events that a therapist would not want to explicate too early.

Arun has a vulnerability associated with needing others and wanting others to see him in a certain way. The therapist would want to start articulating how he sees himself and what he wants to see himself as. The therapist can validate Arun by saying, "It sounds like from what you're saying—and correct me if I'm wrong about this—that it's really important for you to not only just be recognized but also to be held in the kind of esteem you feel you've earned or deserve." The therapist might check with the patient to confirm whether that sounds right to them or if it is a fair statement. Statements like these feel validating to a patient because they capture their phenomenological experience and ease into some of the vulnerabilities that may have come up in the narrative. Otherwise, given that no one can understand at some level, it would feel disappointing when somebody does not recognize that. In sum, a therapist must be careful about validating to prevent validating distortions or being invalidating within their validation because it does not recognize a part of how the patient is feeling.

Knowing when to intervene is not always apparent; however, a therapist must balance the fine line between cutting the patient off, containing them, and giving them room to expand on their concerns, even if it is upsetting. A fishing metaphor can be applied here: One needs to know how much fishing line to let out so the fish can run with the bait before reeling the fish back in. This acts like a choice point that a therapist must grapple with in terms of how much they know of what the patient said versus how much more information the therapist needs before having a sufficient understanding and/or being able to make an intervention. On the basis of the assessment and diagnostic sense, the therapist can determine what they need to do versus how much they need to let the patient tell their story and begin to understand its content and structure. From this point, the therapist must determine what the most empathic approach would be. On the one hand, the therapist does not want the patient to unravel and get too distressed, but on the other hand, the therapist does not want to absolve the patient of necessary stress. Sometimes, people are anxious, which is adaptive, but sometimes, it can exacerbate the situation and become counterproductive. If patients get anxious and therapists absolve them of it too quickly, it essentially lets them know they are unable to tolerate it, which is counterproductive to distress tolerance.

The therapist pays attention to transference reactions. Therapists should keep in mind the quotation, "Don't just do something, sit there." Therapists can sometimes feel pressured into practicing a certain way, but they need to sit and be able to maintain coherent thinking during this arousal or affect storm.

Dialectical Behavior Perspective: Validate Reasonable Fears and Distrust
Effectively working with Arun in this moment necessitates the therapist's ability to actively listen, understand, and empathize with Arun's perspective. It is crucial for the therapist to accurately grasp Arun's confusion regarding the woman's response and his lack of trust in her. Validating his experiences is important to explore the connection between his perceptions and his urge to contact this woman.

Understandably, he finds it challenging to trust someone showing interest in him, considering his history of consistent rejection by peers. Acknowledging and confirming Arun's concerns about potential rejection and recognizing the reasonableness of his mistrust within the context of his invalidating experiences can help him validate his perceptions and emotional responses. By highlighting the validity of his perspective, the therapist fosters self-acceptance and enhances Arun's ability to regulate his emotions. Validation not only strengthens the therapeutic alliance but also promotes the patient's active engagement.

When intervening, the therapist must balance providing acceptance and support with gently guiding the patient toward healthier and more adaptive behaviors. It is akin to riding a teeter-totter, delicately adjusting between conveying acceptance and pushing for change. Achieving the optimal balance requires frequent adjustments to ensure the patient feels understood and validated while also being motivated to make positive changes.

In DBT, the therapist places a strong emphasis on the patient's current emotions. In this case, the therapist's focus would be on helping Arun interrupt his rage and redirect his attention toward increasing awareness and tolerance of underlying vulnerable emotions. Rage is a conditioned response that likely serves as an escape from deeper, painful emotions. Assisting Arun in interrupting his rage and extreme emotional reactions is crucial for him to develop the capacity to tolerate and regulate his underlying vulnerable emotions.

Plan Analysis Perspective: Address the Acceptable Underlying Motive to Foster a Corrective Emotional Experience

The therapist, being mindful that relationship building is still key at this stage of treatment with Arun, would focus on the underlying acceptable motive. By doing this, the therapist may activate the self-healing resources in the patient and work toward more trust in the therapeutic relationship. As such, the motive-oriented therapeutic relationship may be understood as a relationship intervention that sets the stage for a corrective relationship experience, one that the patient likely never experienced throughout his entire life (Arun, on the contrary, experienced much more rejection and traumatic confusion). In this excerpt, Arun's presentation may be underpinned by an activation of plans such as "present as likeable," "be cool," "present as successful" (with the mentioned emotional reaction of pride), and "seek help." Given the slight contradiction in these activated plans, the therapist may say at this point (by trying to be complementary to "seek help"), "I appreciate you asking me for advice and help, and I am willing to help you to sort this out. It sounds like this situation with this girl is something you are proud of and represents some form of success in your personal life. What do you think?" The therapist may pause here to give the patient time to respond, then continue, "It sounds like it is something you were waiting for a long time, and now it is happening. It also means that you don't know what to do and how to interpret her giving you her number, right?" Notice that the therapist does not directly answer the question formulated by the patient ("What do you think?" in the sense of requesting direct reassurance) but focuses on the acceptable underlying motive (while giving the requested reassurance may not necessarily be acceptable in this clinical case).

Like both DBT and TFP perspectives, therapists must find ways to help patients like Arun cope with high arousal. On another level of intervention, a plan analytically informed psychotherapist could focus more on secondary emotions rather than the underlying primary ones that are likely the most painful. This does not mean ignoring or invalidating Arun's underlying primary emotions but determining explicitly the right timing to approach his painful experiences. The therapist is responsible for deciding whether it is a good time to help the patient cope and regulate in the moment or meet the underlying painful affect and work toward change in impulsivity and social interactions, such as Arun's interaction with the woman.

SUMMARY STATEMENT: HOW TO MOVE TOWARD SELF-REFLECTION

This chapter explored several theoretical perspectives on the psychotherapeutic treatment of a patient with high levels of impulsivity and how patients with problems in this functional domain may move toward self-reflectivity.

Research on mechanisms of change that may underlie the psychotherapeutic treatment of impulsive behavior in individuals with personality disorders was reviewed. There is evidence for concluding that change from impulsive behaviors to some kind of patient reflectiveness may act as a mechanism of change in treatments for personality disorders (e.g., Zeifman et al., 2020). The case presentation involved an individual who exhibited high levels of behavioral impulsivity. We independently presented our case formulations based on a description of the case; common and diverse features were discussed.

Several common interventions—ways to address impulsive behaviors and foster a pathway toward self-reflectivity—are essential to the successful treatment of this patient. First, we acknowledge that working with this patient would be challenging, given his propensity to be volatile and aggressive and react with hostility toward others, potentially including the therapist. While developing and maintaining a positive therapeutic alliance is a critical ingredient in all effective therapies (see Chapter 9), it is especially important in treating people with poor impulse control who react with anger or potentially quit treatment prematurely. One shared solution to working with Arun's volatility is engaging him in a collaborative manner and establishing a clear therapeutic frame and focus. Gently interrupting Arun and offering clarification of the meaning of treatment is important. The therapist should avoid assumptions about what the patient wants and instead spend time clarifying the patient's goals. For example, while the therapist may be tempted to assume that Arun wants to control his destructive behaviors, given the serious consequences of these behaviors, it is imperative not to assume that Arun is motivated to change his anger. Defining goals is an excellent way to help Arun take responsibility and ensure that the therapist avoids coming across as controlling. Establishing basic arrangements, including scheduling and the therapist's limits, will also help orient Arun about what to expect and, in turn, regulate his emotional vulnerability.

To promote engagement in treatment and changing maladaptive behaviors, we also emphasized specific therapist attitudes. We stressed that successful treatment of a patient like Arun requires remaining nonjudgmental and validating the grain of logic or reasonableness in the patient's perspective. The therapist can highlight what is reasonable from the patient's perspective by explicitly focusing on the patient's stated goals or implicitly offering a motive-oriented therapeutic relationship. At the same time, the therapist should also tentatively share an alternative perspective that could be true. In doing so, the clinician remains authentic, facilitating Arun's sense of safety in the relationship, and may offer him a new understanding of his situation. The promotion of engagement may benefit from using relationship interventions—for example, interventions consistent with the motive-oriented therapeutic relationship.

With a patient who is impulsive or chronically in an emotionally aroused state, the patient's in-session emotional arousal frequently becomes an important focus. To help the patient engage productively in a therapy session, it is essential that the patient remains within an optimal level of emotional arousal. When emotional arousal is too high, it needs to be the focus of the intervention (see Chapter 4), as also shown in the case of Arun, who repeatedly presented to sessions in an angry state (see the second choice point). We recommend that therapists intervene to assist patients in modulating their affective experiences. This usually means holding off on challenging the patient or actively pursuing change. Instead, it can be more beneficial to intervene with validation and empathy by focusing on the underlying need for help (in the specific situation related to the choice point) or clarifying the patient's in-session experience. The therapist is active—but typically avoids reacting directly to their "countertransferential" urges—in focusing on the patient's unmodulated and often secondary emotions (i.e., anger). The therapist helps the patient become aware of their emotional state and develop more adaptive ways of responding. For example, the therapist can respond by promoting the patient's reflective capacity, mentalizing the interpersonal impact of the patient's actions, or being mindful of in-session emotions in the moment (e.g., "There's a lot of energy in the room right now").

Awareness of impulsive behavior, its precipitants, autobiographical meanings and origins, and consequences in the situation is a hallmark step toward self-reflectivity in the patient. Patients may benefit from a great variety of awareness-fostering routes, including challenging interventions, clarifying, interpreting, developing affect deepening, cognitive restructuring, and reframing. A more fundamental ability in which such new awareness can be embedded is a mindful stance, marked by openness to experience, affect awareness in the moment, and a capacity to observe and regulate emotions and experiences.

Working with angry, impulsive, and emotionally dysregulated patients frequently activates therapists' emotional reactions, and it becomes essential for therapists to modulate their emotions in the situation. Depending on the therapist's framework, they may refer to their own emotional reactions, urges, or countertransference. Therapists need to actively monitor their thoughts, urges, and emotional reactions and work to inhibit unhelpful, counterproductive, and reactive responses. For example, therapists can respond to decrease a patient's emotional arousal by speaking in a calm and measured tone rather than being infected by the patient's heightened emotional state. Of course, we strongly recommend therapists seek supervision, peer support, or their own therapy to clarify personal reactivity and help remain therapeutic in the critical situations facing patients with severe personality difficulties.

Behavioral impulsivity can lead to high-risk and dangerous behaviors, and therapists need to help patients modulate these maladaptive behaviors. This typically requires helping patients identify the triggers to their behaviors and recognize the (sometimes dramatic) consequences of their actions. It may require dialectical strategies, responding by balancing a focus on interrupting maladaptive behaviors with a focus on validation and empathy because too strong a push for change can trigger defensiveness and anger. The therapist can highlight, clarify, and validate patients' experiences while helping them consider alternate ways of perceiving and reacting to a situation.

In sum, although our conceptual lenses differ, the three case formulations and recommended interventions share more commonalities than differences. Points of divergence are mostly limited to theoretical terms (e.g., defenses vs. coping vs. emotional escape behaviors) rather than emphasizing understanding the case and intervening at specific choice points. As noted, the shared common emphases included a focus on the patient's in-session emotional arousal; the provision of therapist relational attributes, including nonjudgment, validation, and genuineness to build and strengthen the patient's engagement; the promotion of awareness of the behavior underlying nonproblematic motives; strategies to facilitate awareness of the triggers of behavioral impulsivity; the promotion of awareness of the interpersonal consequences of dysregulated states; and focus on eliminating and controlling impulsive behavior symptoms (i.e., aggressive outbursts).

8

MOVING FROM COGNITIVE-PERCEPTUAL DISTURBANCES TO COHERENT AND REALITY-BASED NARRATIVES

This chapter explores the functional domain of cognitive–perceptual impairments, including psychotic symptoms in personality pathology, and examines how to help patients develop a coherent narrative that is anchored in reality. It also looks at how to address and effectively interrupt dissociative states and develop a more solid sense of self-identity.

To the best of our knowledge, there is little empirical research on the treatment of cognitive disturbances in patients with personality pathology, and there is little empirical research demonstrating that shifts in cognitive disturbances are a mechanism of change in psychotherapy for personality disorders. This chapter, therefore, does not include an extended discussion of empirical support as in previous chapters. Limited research on other clinical populations indicates that narrative cohesiveness predicts symptom change (Angus et al., 2017, 2019; Boritz et al., 2017). Using the Narrative-Emotion Process Coding System (NEPCS 2.0; Angus et al., 2017), Kramer, Simonini, et al. (2023) demonstrated for a sample of 57 patients with borderline personality disorder (BPD) undergoing brief psychiatric treatment that the reduction of problematic narrative markers (i.e., empty storytelling and same-old storytelling) and

https://doi.org/10.1037/0000388-009
Understanding Mechanisms of Change in Psychotherapies for Personality Disorders, by U. Kramer, K. N. Levy, and S. McMain

the increase of so-called transition markers (i.e., reflective and experiential storytelling) early in the therapy process predicted symptom reduction. On the basis of our elaborations in Chapter 2, we speculate that for many individuals with personality disorders, modifying repetitive problematic patterns of cognitive disturbances is a key process accounting for the effectiveness of psychotherapy.

We begin by describing the case of Irene, a patient who presented with cognitive disturbances and dissociation.[1] We offer our diagnostic impressions and a case formulation from three different psychotherapeutic perspectives—dialectical behavior therapy (DBT), transference-focused psychotherapy (TFP), and plan analysis—comparing areas of overlap and differences. This discussion is followed by considering how best to intervene at three specific choice points in therapy. We then elaborate on how a therapist can help the patient move from rigid delusional beliefs to a more reality-based narrative and improve the patient's ability to engage in rational decision making, helping her synthesize a dichotomous view of herself and others. The chapter concludes with a summary of our recommended interventions that aim to help the patient move toward a coherent and reality-based narrative. The case of Irene is used to highlight general principles that may apply to other individuals with severe cognitive–perceptual disturbance.

THE CASE OF IRENE

This case was selected for analysis in this chapter because the patient's behavior is characterized by highly unusual thoughts, moments of cognitive confusion, and dissociation.

Irene is a 28-year-old woman who had never previously sought help for psychological problems. She presented as intelligent and hardworking, with a university degree in social work. Since graduating 3 years ago, she began multiple jobs and quit each within 3 months, leaving herself without any substantial professional experience. During the first session, she was accompanied by her mother, who did most of the talking, while Irene remained mostly silent. The mother, an accomplished woman in her 60s, who had run a successful marketing company from a young age, burst into tears at the onset of the session and spoke of the suffering her daughter was causing her. She emphasized that she wanted only the best for Irene, and the fact that Irene was not working and had no professional ambition caused her great distress. Clearly,

---

[1]The case of Irene and other cases presented throughout this chapter has been modified to disguise the patients' identities and protect their confidentiality.

career success was important to the mother, and Irene's current profile and psychological problems were at odds with some of the family's values and expectations.

Irene is an only child of parents engaged in high-profile careers in academia and management. She described herself as having been a timid child with few friends and explained that this was because she lacked interest in socializing. As a child, she enjoyed reading, writing, and solitary activities such as computer games and handicrafts. She described her childhood as happy and mentioned that she spent most of her time on her own, which she found refreshing and relaxing.

When asked about her father, Irene remained silent. She mentioned that her relationship with him had been "odd" and that, at times, there was no relationship because he was always away at work. Irene denied any history of physical or sexual abuse and, at the same time, made a cryptic remark about her father when she stated, "I am unable to say something about my father that would be untruthful." On further inquiry, she stated she felt betrayed and let down by him, even though he was currently paying for all her living expenses. Importantly, there was no evidence of sexual abuse in Irene's history. She reported that she had never had a lasting romantic relationship due to her "need to be alone."

Over the last 3 years, Irene had started and quit a new job at least 10 times, the shortest period of employment lasting just 1 week. She explained that her reason for leaving in each case was due to bullying at the workplace. She had always felt that social work was her calling, and she began each job with high hopes, but her motivation to work rapidly deteriorated once she began working. Every new job seemed to follow the same pattern. From the start, she was meticulous and eager to do things right. Thereafter, she would feel overwhelmed by new tasks that felt beyond her capabilities. She described how she would work "night and day" to "get it right" and would successfully master new skills within a few days or weeks. In contrast to her colleagues, she felt she was working "perfectly." Yet, from her perspective, her colleagues would quickly begin to pick on her. For example, she recounted others making snide comments such as "You're very motivated" or "It's good to have someone so effective here." In Irene's mind, these were thinly disguised attacks on her. Consequently, she felt increasingly isolated at work and stopped socializing with colleagues; she avoided people by working from home when possible. When Irene described her last work experience as "traumatic," her mother encouraged her to pursue psychotherapy. In addition to the typical pattern of first assuming others disliked her and then avoiding them, at her last workplace, she was convinced that five female colleagues were plotting against her and had created a public website designed to put her down and out her as a lesbian. Irene was uncertain about her sexual orientation. On one occasion, she told her therapist that the purported website claimed she was a sex worker. There was no evidence of such a website.

When Irene described her version of these events, she became emotionally dysregulated, and her discourse became hard to follow. Her thoughts were suggestive of her losing control: "People are doing things to me. I may be harmed. I am powerless to deal with them." She quickly became confused about the time, location, and people, making it extremely difficult for the therapist to make sense of the narrative. The therapist repeatedly intervened to ask for clarification.

In a semistructured diagnostic interview, Irene's clinical presentation was consistent with a diagnosis of paranoid personality disorder. Other personality disorders (particularly borderline and narcissistic) were identified as differential diagnoses. There was no indication of childhood trauma; however, Irene did not provide enough information to completely rule out a trauma history. Because she reported no self-harming behaviors, impulsive acts, or suicidal thoughts, an emergent psychotic disorder was ruled out. From a dimensional perspective, Irene rated high on psychoticism and negative affectivity and low on agreeableness.

CASE FORMULATION: ASSESSING COGNITIVE-PERCEPTUAL DISTURBANCES

Case formulation is the basis for making meaning of complex and, at times, ambiguous clinical information and provides a framework for intervention. We begin by considering how to conceptualize Irene's apparent cognitive–perceptual disturbances and how they manifest in therapy sessions. Given the severe cognitive disturbances, we begin by discussing our diagnostic impressions.

Dialectical Behavior Formulation: Explore Past Trauma and Invalidation

In DBT, the process of case formulation begins with an initial assessment aimed at understanding the origins and maintenance of the patient's difficulties. In Irene's case, it is important to explore how her social environment and potential biological vulnerability factors may be interconnected with her pathology. A comprehensive understanding of these factors can inform the development of more targeted and effective clinical interventions.

Given Irene's mistrust of others, avoidance of relationships, and engagement in dissociative behaviors, as well as her evident challenges in her relationship with her father and reluctance to discuss it, it becomes crucial for the therapist to investigate the presence of any invalidating and traumatic experiences in her life. The dynamics within her relationship with her father raise questions about the potential presence of traumatic invalidation, which could be an underlying factor contributing to her symptoms and overall difficulties. The nature of her relationship with her father raises questions about the possible traumatic invalidation that may underlie her symptoms. While Irene denied any history of physical or sexual abuse and, at the same time, made a cryptic remark about her father when she stated, "I am unable to say something about my father that would be untruthful," it is possible that she may be reluctant to share any traumatic material with the therapist and, over time, as the relationship with the therapist strengthens, more details may emerge. The therapist can inquire more about the nature of the relationship with the father; however, this inquiry should be done with caution. Given her fragile sense of self and identity problems, this patient may be highly suggestible, and it is prudent to avoid leading her or saying something to contribute to implanting a false memory. Further diagnostic assessment is required to determine if Irene meets the criteria for complex trauma in addition to her personality pathology.

Irene's symptoms, such as dissociation, incoherent narrative, mistrust of others, avoidance of relationships, aggressive behavior, and emotional instability, may be adaptive responses to her environment. These symptoms align with a trauma reaction, even if Irene denies any history of sexual or physical abuse. It is important to acknowledge that significant invalidating experiences can contribute to traumatic reactions.

Irene's symptom profile suggests deficits in emotion regulation, and her behaviors appear to be a way to modulate intense and distressing emotions. For instance, her dissociative behavior may function as a means to escape from painful emotional memories. Similarly, her avoidance of relationships, long working hours, and efforts to avoid making errors could be strategies to steer clear of situations that trigger memories of invalidating relationships.

If Irene's dissociation and relationship difficulties are connected to her traumatic invalidation history, it becomes crucial to address these traumatic experiences in treatment. It is essential to create a therapeutic focus that includes exploring and processing the traumatic events, taking into account Irene's potential distress associated with them.

Transference-Focused Formulation: Differentiating Complex PTSD From Borderline Personality Disorder

From a TFP perspective, in accordance with the need for diagnostic clarity, we again assume the possibility of complex trauma. If this patient is identity diffused, there are concerns regarding her suggestibility. From an empirical viewpoint, the differential diagnosis between complex posttraumatic stress disorder (CPTSD), which stems from childhood abuse, and BPD is important, but only a handful of studies (e.g., Cloitre et al., 2014) have investigated this with a rigorous lens. Many researchers focusing on CPTSD may assume that BPD is CPTSD and not a separate diagnostic category. However, there is strong empirical support for BPD and CPTSD being distinct conditions. In a randomized controlled trial for the treatment of PTSD that enrolled 280 women, Cloitre et al. (2014) conducted a latent class analysis to distinguish participants with BPD, PTSD, and CPTSD. The researchers found patients with BPD to be more disruptive than the other two subgroups and even considered excluding them from the trial. The question they faced was whether it was possible to differentiate patients with BPD and those with CPTSD, and the analysis showed that these presentations differed considerably. The following symptoms predicted the likelihood of a BPD diagnosis: frantic efforts to avoid abandonment, an unstable sense of self, unstable and intense interpersonal relationships, and impulsivity. In contrast, patients with CPTSD presented with clinical features that were more consistent with extreme manifestations of anxiety disorders and did not show the BPD manifestations. They had more self-evaluations (and not identity diffusion) and presented with avoidance in relationships, as if their greatest fear was related to getting hurt in a relationship, which differs from the stormy relationships seen in BPD. Furthermore, they did not present with as many self-harming or suicidal behaviors as the patients with BPD. For clinical purposes, the implications of these conclusions may not be as clear-cut, but they may help us make the correct diagnosis for someone like Irene.

The findings may be useful in clarifying the nature of the self-presentation in the case of Irene. Is her identity diffused, as in BPD, or is her negative sense of self related to an anxiety disorder and depression? What is the nature of her relationships? Is she afraid of getting hurt, thus avoiding relationships, or are her symptoms more chaotic? Individuals diagnosed with BPD will often vacillate between an attraction to relationships and pushing away from them. Irene's absence of self-injurious behavior is more consistent with CPTSD than BPD.

Another open diagnostic question is how "psychotic"—or how distant from a shared perception of reality—is this patient? Are the cognitive problems quasi-psychotic (Zanarini et al., 1990), transient, and related to interpersonal stressors (American Psychiatric Association, 2022) or prodromal, in the sense of an emergent psychotic disorder (American Psychiatric Association, 2022)? Differential diagnoses to consider include paranoid personality disorder and schizotypal personality disorder. In terms of personality organization, we can ask whether Irene is someone who is organized at a psychotic level but functions at a borderline level or if she is someone who is organized at a borderline level and sometimes dips into a psychotic level of functioning.

We mentioned earlier that Irene commented, "I am unable to say something about my father that would be untruthful." This offers an opportunity for the therapist to seek clarification—for example, "You say you can't say anything negative or untruthful about your father, but most people, even if they had good parents whom they loved, might still find something negative about them. What makes it so difficult for you to say anything about your father, specifically something negative about him?" Irene may be concerned that if she said something negative, it would make her a "bad person." It could be the same dynamic she has regarding her sexuality. In conclusion, from a TFP perspective, and more generally, the differential diagnosis of complex trauma needs to be clarified in this case. Also, Irene's cognitive–perceptual problems should be explored more deeply, and the question of a psychotic personality organization versus borderline personality organization (Kernberg, 1984) remains open.

Plan Analysis Formulation: In-Session Behaviors as Avoidance Plans

From a plan analysis perspective, after the more formal diagnostic clarification (as described in the TFP formulation), it would be helpful to observe and explain some of this patient's peculiar in-session behaviors. These behaviors may be underpinned by a number of avoidance plans that may explain the quasi-psychotic content or otherwise dysregulated behavior. These may involve plans such as "avoid opening up or engaging with this therapist," "avoid showing any weakness," and "avoid being hurt by others." Plans such as "show the other that you are able to respond quickly and swiftly," "show that you are strong, in charge, and intelligent," "attack the other" (to "protect yourself and your boundaries"), and "make up bizarre stories" are active and highly problematic for Irene's relationships.

In contrast to many other patients, Irene does not seem to use plans to foster incoherent presentations of the self to attract attention, but it looks like she does quite the opposite. She seems to adopt a peculiar interpersonal cognitively and perceptively incoherent stance to give the other a clear message: "Back off!" While these behaviors seem to convey an implicit message to her interaction partners that she needs to be left alone, the therapist may observe that she is suffering due to her peculiar interaction style. Irene's distress is substantiated by her coming to therapy (even without her mother's push, which may be explained by a plan such as "get healed," or "do everything to get out of this difficult financial situation"). The problem with the notion of suffering at this point is that it may not be conceivable in Irene's current concept of self that she may need help. She dismisses her father in a narrative presenting herself as feeling betrayed by him while still needing his financial support to survive. A similar contradiction may activate in the therapeutic interaction with the therapist. There seems to be a need for help (i.e., the patient continues to come to therapy), but this concept of neediness is so distressing to her, reminding her of boundary-overstepping interaction experiences with other caretakers in her life, that the only way for her to interact is to use incoherent language to fill the therapy hour to try to keep the therapist at bay.

From a motive-oriented therapeutic relationship viewpoint, this patient's presentation is particularly complex because of conflicting underlying plans. To be appropriately responsive to this patient's presentation, the therapist would need to (a) express the importance of respecting boundaries between the patient and therapist (both physically and emotionally, which is complementary to the patient's central plan "protect yourself and your boundaries") while, at the same time, (b) underlining that there may be aspects Irene would need help with, which could thus be complementary to the patient's equally central plan, "do everything to get out of this difficult situation." The latter could be explored at this early stage of therapy.

In conclusion, from a plan analysis case formulation perspective, the cognitive problems in Irene's case may be due to a conflict between experience structures or semantic nodes ("plans") from her biography, in that the patient aims to protect herself by inventing harmful and incoherent stories to keep others at bay and pursuing better mental health, being mindful of the current limitations in her life.

Toward a Common Formulation

Synthesizing our three perspectives, we agree on three major points, while a few aspects are open for discussion. First, we agree that in addition to the patient's personality disorder, we must consider the possibility of traumatic invalidating experiences in the patient's childhood, leaving her with important barriers to engaging in constructive interpersonal relationships and the development of a coherent sense of self. Second, we agree that there is a need to clarify more about Irene's developmental history and use all the information (verbal and nonverbal) offered by her to understand more about her inner life and experiences. Third, we observe avoidance behaviors (or avoidance plans) that are highly rigid and so pervasive that they also affect the consistency of Irene's narrative and overall manner. There is agreement that it is important to work toward interrupting avoidance behaviors, increasing the patient's sense of safety through the therapeutic relationship, and focus on transforming maladaptive underlying cognitive–emotional processes.

The focus on the invalidating context may partially contradict the more in-session observations in the other formulation approaches. Also, the degree to which emotional and representational processes are central to understanding the cognitive–perceptual disturbance in personality disorders may differ for each case formulation approach.

CHOICE POINTS AND OPPORTUNITIES FOR CHANGE

Three clinical excerpts that illustrate crucial choice points in the treatment of Irene are presented in this section. We discuss how to intervene from our different treatment perspectives at these three choice points. First, we discuss how to address the delusional beliefs underpinning Irene's clinical presentation. Second, we discuss the possible pathways to helping Irene make more informed and rational choices in her daily life. Third, we discuss the integration of opposing or dichotomous views of the self and others. Fourth, we consider how and why we maintain a productive emotion focus with this patient, which we believe is relevant to all three choice points. Table 8.1 synthesizes generic and approach-specific strategies that therapists might use and relevant patient processes in the three choice points presented in this chapter.

"There Is This Website Created by My Colleagues With the Intent to Harm Me": Targeting Delusional Beliefs

Irene's statement about a website she claims discusses her sexuality publicly—in which five female colleagues were "plotting" against her to portray her as a "lesbian"—seemed delusional. Neither we nor Irene were able to find any evidence that such a website exists. Her belief appeared to be an example of quasi-psychotic content or a strong transient belief related to stress triggered by an interpersonal situation. Once the interpersonal stress wanes, the belief subsides. Irene temporarily lost touch with reality in circumscribed ways that pertain to her sexuality. She showed no signs of a fixed delusion. Her claim that her colleagues created a website suggests that she perceives others as threatening. This does not rule out the possibility that it could ultimately become a long-standing delusion; the current presentation is in reaction to an interpersonal situation. After quitting the job and escaping from her colleagues, she made little mention of the website.

TABLE 8.1. How to Foster a Path Toward a Coherent and Reality-Based Narrative

Generic therapist interventions	Specific therapist interventions	Patient processes
Choice point: Addressing delusional belief		
• Build a therapeutic relationship and convey genuine interest. • Increase emotional awareness. • Maintain an emotion focus.	• Promote awareness of arousal. • Identify triggers. • Foster emotional awareness.	• Transform beliefs. • Decrease in-session emotional arousal. • Increase awareness of situational triggers. • Increase emotional awareness and acceptance.
Choice point: Addressing irrational behaviors		
• Manage risk. • Promote self-awareness. • Focus on motivation to change.	• Assess risk to self and others. • Confront the patient with risk. • Promote awareness of wisdom. • Avoid polarization. • Highlight the freedom to choose. • Maintain an emotion focus.	• Become aware of real risk. • Increase impulse control. • Strengthen authentic self-presentation. • Understand the impact of one's behavior. • Increase emotional awareness and acceptance.
Choice point: Addressing opposing views		
• Promote awareness in the patient.	• Differentiate between real and false self-presentation. • Highlight contradictory views.	• Increase awareness of aspects of the self. • Increase awareness of opposing views about the self and others. • Increase awareness and tolerance of different perspectives of the self.

Plan Analysis Perspective: Initially Accept the Claim as True for Relationship Purposes

From a plan analysis perspective, a therapist may initially respond by taking Irene's concerns seriously, as if the website does exist. For example, they might say, "This is really concerning. Let's have a look together. Where is this website? If there is nothing there yet, is there any proposal or content we could look at together? Can you bring that material to the session next week?" This response may help build the therapeutic relationship and complement several plans previously discussed in the plan analytic case formulation. It is important for the therapist to appear genuinely concerned about Irene's claim that her colleagues are publicly making false statements about her sexuality to avoid a possibly invalidating experience for the patient. In response to these inquiries, the patient may acknowledge that she has no evidence of the website's existence. Relevant to the diagnosis of a more transient psychotic state, Irene may consider the evidence herself rather than having the therapist directly present counterevidence for the delusion. After she considers the facts, the contradictions, and the reality of the situation, the quasipsychotic content may dissipate.

Dialectical Behavior Perspective: Create Distance From Paranoid Thoughts

Several approaches can be effective in responding to Irene in this particular moment. A crucial initial step is to help Irene engage in reflection and examine her thoughts before attempting to modify them. The therapist can facilitate this by reflecting on Irene's thoughts and encouraging her to elaborate on her comments regarding the website. This would allow Irene to gain some distance from her thoughts and start observing them as mere thoughts. Through this process, a closer examination of her thoughts can help differentiate between facts and assumptions. For instance, Irene may clarify that she never witnessed or heard people discussing the website. Irene can gradually become aware that her fearful thoughts are recurring patterns triggered by predictable cues potentially related to traumatic and invalidating memories.

It is important to recognize that Irene's paranoid thoughts indicate heightened emotional arousal and perceived threat, which can compromise her cognitive processes. Thoughts are more likely to be extreme and distorted when individuals are emotionally aroused. Engaging in rumination about the website would likely exacerbate her emotional arousal and reinforce her cognitive distortions. Therefore, another intervention strategy is to help Irene reduce her emotional arousal to think more clearly and rationally about the situation. The therapist might respond by acknowledging Irene's intense emotional state and its impact on her breathing, saying, "It seems like your emotions are really intense right now, and it's difficult to catch your breath." This remark increases Irene's mindfulness of her emotional state and breathing, taking a step toward emotion modulation. If Irene acknowledges the extremity of her emotional arousal and expresses motivation to reduce it, the therapist can guide her in specific distress tolerance skills such as deep breathing or progressive muscle relaxation.

Once Irene's emotional arousal has de-escalated, she can be collaboratively engaged in a behavior chain analysis of this situation to better understand what prompted her reaction and the links between her emotions and distorted thoughts. The therapist can help Irene identify a specific internal or external event that triggered her sense of threat and paranoid thoughts. The content of Irene's thoughts suggests she feels out of control, unsafe, and powerless to do anything (i.e., "People are doing things to me. I may be harmed. I am powerless to deal with them"). This critical information provides a window into what underlies Irene's response. It may be that through an intensive analysis of this in-session moment, the therapist can help Irene identify the emotional drivers underlying her communications about the threatening situation.

Throughout the therapy process, the therapist can work with Irene to increase her awareness of the repetitive nature of her distorted thoughts, the triggers that activate them, and the unpleasant emotions that accompany them. It is important to emphasize the acceptance of her primary emotional experiences and enhance her ability to tolerate these emotions. In addition, a focus should be placed on assisting Irene in transforming her maladaptive emotional responses through exposure exercises and reinforcing behaviors that are opposite to her predominant emotions.

Transference-Focused Perspective: Grounding the Patient and Addressing Psychotic Episodes

From a TFP perspective, while many of the previous ideas would be considered acceptable, they sound a bit technical. To illustrate how a TFP therapist might work with Irene to directly target her delusional beliefs, we cite some experiences with two other patients. In one case, that of a male patient with a profile similar to Irene's, the therapist confronted him about his quasi-psychotic content in a gentle way by listening to what he was saying, clarifying things he said, and bringing into his awareness the spared aspects in an effort to understand the full clinical presentation. The other case was a female patient who required crisis intervention due to recurrent delusional states. In one instance, the patient had a psychotic episode in session, saying she was seeing fire coming out of the sockets in the wall and talking in ways the therapist could not follow. Before starting a TFP program, the patient had been in a DBT program, which was helpful to her and described by her as similar to TFP. This patient benefitted from the therapist being aware that she would enter a transient psychotic state every time she was angry, which would happen frequently. Grounding the patient in her emotions helped calm her down and move her out of the psychotic state. Sometimes, the only solution for some patients may be to hospitalize them to help calm them down. While we agree that we want to do everything possible to avoid hospitalization, it may not always be avoidable in transient psychotic cases. It would be important for Irene to have occasions for gentle reality testing, increasing her awareness of reality.

"I Want to Be a Sex Worker": Helping the Patient Make Realistic, Rational Life Choices

The second choice point and opportunity for change appeared when the patient discussed her professional goals and how to earn her living.

> I want to be a sex worker. You know, my career has been a catastrophe for now, so someone advised me, and she is right, that I should change jobs. Social work has been a failure for me, but I have all that's needed to make men, also women [*in an insistent tone of voice*] happy. So, I want to enter the sex work business. I am serious! I want to be—you know what it is like. I want to undergo that intensive training to become a prostitute, and I want to start now. Do you know where I can get information? This is so important for me. The best thing I can offer to society is my body, and if they turn me down, I will strip down in front of them and show what I can do! [*Irene gets up, makes movements to undress, and quickly sits down in the chair again, interrupting her behavior.*]

Here, the concern is how to help Irene avoid making impulsive decisions in favor of rational and informed ones. Decisions about what profession she wants to practice, where she wants to live, where she wants to work, and what type of relationships she wants are big life choices. At age 28, Irene was still financially dependent on her parents, but they announced they would end their support 6 months later. How can long-term goals influence the patient's decisions at a given moment? Irene's statement about wanting to be a sex worker appears to be an impulsive and irrational reflection possibly leading to a harmful decision. She ultimately did not act on this decision but still threatened to move forward with it. The challenge for the therapist is how to help her move toward a more emotionally balanced decision.

Transference-Focused Perspective: Shifting From Being Neutral to Offering Guidance

From a TFP perspective, the therapist may want to better understand what lies beneath this comment. The first step is to clarify: "Can you say more about this?" It is usually best to adopt a technically neutral stance by remaining at an equal distance from the patient's perspectives of the conflict and taking a nonjudgmental stance with respect to the comment. However, it may be necessary to deviate from technical neutrality at times, especially if the patient seems likely to carry out the threatened behavior. In that situation, it is best to acknowledge the patient's impulse, offer some direction, and then explore this direction together. This is illustrated in another clinical example. A male patient, George, came in one day, furiously angry about something that had happened at work. He said he was being picked on by some coworkers. George was intelligent but peculiar and tended to be ostracized by others, which is much like Irene's schizotypal narcissistic-paranoid presentation. When he became angry at his coworkers, he would harbor a revenge fantasy about how he would expose them as the corrupt individuals they were. It was clear that putting this plan into action would get him fired, and George's desire was not truly to expose others but rather to resolve his current situation. The therapist realized it was time to break from technical neutrality: "Look, George, I understand how your coworkers are making you feel, and I can certainly understand the impulse to retaliate. But I am afraid that if you acted on your urges, you'd end up getting fired and put a lot of your gains at risk." The aim of this intervention was to help the patient distinguish between reality and internal fantasy. Humans fantasize all the time but usually do not act on their fantasies. Most people understand the difference between their internal world and the external reality; some individuals, like George, do not.

In Irene's case, it may be advisable to explore her thinking more. Although the therapist is not worried that Irene is going to become a sex worker, at least not immediately, it is necessary to explore further and see how well-articulated her plan is. In George's case, there was genuine concern that he might enact his revenge fantasy the next day, so it was important for the therapist to acknowledge that fantasies are okay and need to be understood because they tell us something about ourselves and what we want. For Irene, it may also be helpful to break technical neutrality: "Look, I want to understand more about your interest in being a sex worker because I think it's important to discuss it further before you make a decision. Ultimately, you are an adult, and you will make your own decision about what to do." If there is a risk of Irene acting on this plan before the next session, it would be advisable to attempt to get her to agree to continue discussing it first, giving her time to explore. If it turns out that her plan is real, it would be advisable to raise awareness of the dangerous consequences of such a choice, such as sexually transmissible infections, the risk of violence, and so forth. The therapist may want to say, "You know, as you explain more about your interest in doing this, I can understand what you think it would provide in terms of freedom of expression [or other content]. However, on another level, there are some serious risks associated with it. I wonder what your thoughts are about those." It would be important to see if the patient understands the risks. She might be dismissive of them (e.g., "I don't think those are going to be problems"), or she might acknowledge them. In the latter case, if the concern is truly coming from the patient rather than imposed by the therapist, it can be explored. The therapist could introduce the metaphor of a clock—for example, "Is that something we need to deal with immediately or is it something we can unpack and explore later?" The metaphor of the clock, or the good time of any therapeutic intervention, may help to understand what the therapist should do when facing the patient.

Dialectical Behavior Perspective: Distinguishing the Emotional Mind and the Wise Mind

In this situation, several DBT interventions can be applied to address Irene's risky behaviors and prevent their recurrence. The therapist's initial focus would be to assess whether Irene's desire to become a sex worker aligns with her long-term goals and values or if it is an impulsive expression amid intense emotions. To help Irene differentiate between an "emotional mind" statement and a "wise mind" statement, the therapist can encourage her to observe her current state of mind. An emotional mind state is characterized by intense emotions and impulsive actions without considering the consequences, whereas a wise mind state involves being aware of one's feelings and goals and responding calmly and in a goal-directed manner. The therapist can prompt Irene by asking, "When you mention wanting to be a sex worker, do you recognize which state of mind you're in? Is this decision driven by your emotional mind, or is it a reasonable and wise-mind decision? What would your wise mind say?" By guiding Irene to reflect on her state of mind, she can gain emotional distance from her thoughts and feelings, leading to improved emotional regulation and more rational decision making and behavior.

If Irene acknowledges that she is emotionally overwhelmed, the therapeutic goal would be to help her prevent impulsive behaviors stemming from this state. If the risk of impulsive action is high at that moment, the therapist can express concern about the potential consequences of making significant decisions while in an emotional mind state. For example, the therapist might express worry by saying, "I'm concerned that deciding to become a sex worker when you're in an emotional mind state could lead to regrets later on." The therapist can then encourage Irene to shift into a wise-mind state by slowing down, regulating her emotions, and refraining from making any major decisions. Ultimately, by assisting Irene in modulating her emotions and reducing arousal, the therapist can enable her to become more aware of her emotional needs and make adaptive choices.

If there are indications that Irene is genuinely serious about her intentions and the risk of acting impulsively is high, the therapist should prioritize preventing the impulsive behavior and helping Irene step back to make a decision from a more grounded state of mind. The therapist can directly, nonjudgmentally, and authentically address the behavior, stating their concerns and potential negative outcomes. For instance, the therapist might say, "It strikes me as a rather extreme approach to making money." The therapist can also engage in self-disclosure, expressing their reaction to Irene's plan: "I'm concerned that if you decide to engage in sex work, it might ultimately leave you feeling worse about yourself."

Alternatively, on the basis of Irene's tone and quality of voice, the therapist might assess that her statement is conveyed in a dramatic manner and she has no real intention of acting on it. In this case, the therapist can explore the underlying meaning behind the statement. This exploration could involve a direct inquiry: "Do you genuinely want to become a sex worker, or is something else going on beneath that comment?" The therapist could also employ a dialectical response in an irreverent manner, aiming to provoke a shift in Irene's perspective. For example, the therapist might playfully extend the patient's statement by asking, "So, have you started advertising your services?"

Plan Analysis Perspective: Informing the Patient While Promoting Autonomy

According to the plan analysis formulation outlined earlier, it may be important to adopt a mixed intervention strategy. The first thing to do would be to mark the big decision Irene is about to make and the potential dramatics of its implications. The therapist may reflect on whether that decision should be taken lightly, putting more time into the decision itself. On the basis of the case formulation, we can also understand Irene's statement in the context of her plans as the expression of something important. This expression may distract the therapist from other, more relevant content (e.g., the fact that she will have a financial problem when her parents stop supporting her, which is related to her becoming a sex worker to solve this problem). Alternatively, expressing the wish to work as a prostitute may interpersonally test what would happen if she threatened to do so as a consequence of her parents withdrawing their financial support. This may be a relationship test to clarify whether her parents would continue to stand with her if she started working in the sex business. Finally, it could also be that this patient is hinting at unresolved body-related issues, such as abuse, in the past. These speculations would have to be clarified in further assessments.

According to such a formulation, this statement is a possible opening into a relationship crisis. Such an expression may indicate that the patient expects the therapist to impose their vision on her, that she expects the therapist— like many others—to give well-intentioned advice to not engage in sex work. By marking her statement, "I want to be a sex worker," as dramatic, it may imply that it is dangerous or potentially negative. Thus, it is important to find the right formulation that is not playing into the patient's expected responses from the other. Given the case formulation, the most important component seems to be working toward Irene's underlying acceptable plans, those related to staying in control and deciding what kind of work she ultimately wants to do. If this formulation is correct, the optimal therapist response should be, "You, dear patient, will decide."

If it is true that some of Irene's central plans are related to staying in control of things, including her decisions, the patient may calm down after such an intervention. If this happens, it remains an open question whether Irene can contain or regulate her emotional reaction to such an intervention and make good use of it. In this situation, it may ultimately be a clinical decision by the therapist. If the therapist notices an action tendency within themselves informing them that "You (as the therapist) should be making that decision" (e.g., the therapist feels pressured to make the decision for Irene), it becomes clear that there is an interpersonal-instrumental component to this statement. The latter should then be taken into account in the intervention. At this point, it is, of course, important for the therapist not to act on this action tendency but address the patient's underlying motive for stating her action tendency to make an impulsive decision. Here, the therapist should respect Irene's space and assume that her capacity for making wise decisions is preserved. The therapist, focusing on the underlying motive, might say, "It sounds like you are about to make a big decision in your life, right? One important thing I want to tell you is that, ultimately, it will be your decision. Whatever you decide, you will own that decision, carry it forward, and make it work. Can you tell me more about what makes you so dissatisfied with social work?"

This observation also enriches the understanding of Irene's personality functioning and, ultimately, the case formulation. The therapist may wonder what kind of experiences Irene has had to make her so sensitive that other people could impose their opinions or decisions on her—that people could make a decision for her about a dramatic career shift. From her history, we know that her father seemed to have a say in her decision to become a social worker and that Irene does not seem to make her own decisions and may never have made a major decision herself. This may also involve decisions about with whom she wants to live or how she wants to make money. As mentioned earlier, this challenge may be related to her difficulty with being connected to her innermost wishes and emotions in the moment, connected to "What do I need here? Do I want to be here or somewhere else? Do I want to do this? Where do I go in life?" These problems may be related to fundamental "alienation," a feature described in severe forms of personality disorders (Sachse, 2020). These open questions should be clarified to help Irene learn from this process of decision making to develop a deep connection with herself and the ability to make her own decisions in the future.

Another Transference-Focused Perspective: Using Irreverent Statements
While this may not necessarily be the right moment, irreverent statements may also be used in certain moments of therapy. Without expressing it, we might have had an irreverent thought when reading that Irene was a social worker: "Well, that is one way of being a social worker!" Again, we would not necessarily share this comment with Irene at this stage, but it is important to attend to and reflect on our reactions to what patients say or how they present. Using irreverence may be another way of being authentic, and consideration of one's reaction may provide important insights into how others experience the patient in addition to one's own experience of the patient. Although it may not be useful to express one's countertransference to the patient, it can aid understanding. What is needed in this case is understanding Irene's behavior as asserting that she wants to do something, perhaps something that would provoke her family. She said she expected a reaction from not only the therapist but also other people. Such an intervention might allow this patient to make a more conscious decision about what she wants to do. Ultimately, she might recognize that her impulse to begin sex work represents her desire to provoke her parents. Her parents, who would love for her to live at home and pursue social work, would see this as a big "screw you." This interpretation may also indicate that she cannot say something negative about her father, yet she wants to send him a big "screw you," possibly in response to something negative that she may not be able to acknowledge.

"You Also Have a Personality Disorder!": Fostering Integration Between Opposing Views of Self and Others

This choice point deals with integrating dichotomous or opposing views of the self and others. The third excerpt is from Session 8, in which the therapist discussed the results from the semistructured interview that yielded a symptom presentation consistent with a paranoid personality disorder and linked this diagnosis to Irene's experiences and behavior. The therapist avoided referring to a specific *Diagnostic and Statistical Manual of Mental Disorders* category because of the unclear differential diagnosis and the potential harm to the relationship when talking overtly about "paranoid personality disorder" at this point. The therapist communicated the diagnosis in a careful and behavior-oriented way, avoiding giving just a label, summarizing what had been observed, and referring to "personality disorder" as commonly used in medical language. It was difficult for Irene to hear this, and she interrupted in a cognitively and affectively dysregulated manner with the following:

> So there it is. I have a personality disorder. What the fuck! Nobody, [*yelling*] nobody has ever told me this! This is fake! You are fake! Everything you do and say is fake. And one thing: If I have a personality disorder, it is because of you only. You made me sick with your nonsense. And here I am now, discussing this nonsense with you. By the way, you also have a personality disorder! So, you know it. That's all I have to say!

Clarification-Oriented Perspective: Reformulating Attacks Via Motives

From a clarification-oriented psychotherapy viewpoint (Sachse, 2020), Irene's attacking behavior toward the therapist and its apparent contradiction to her more authentic search for help in this context can be understood from an interaction maneuver, or game, perspective. Irene's activated motive is that she is expressing a need for help, which is also consistent with what the therapist observes. Objectively, her father will cut off her financial support in a few months, and she needs to find a solution for her professional life and resolve the impact of her psychological problems on her personal life. The therapist may formulate a contradiction between underlying motives (i.e., related to being recognized as a person and as someone who fundamentally wishes to get better) and transparent interaction maneuvers in the therapy relationship (i.e., her attack on the therapist). The therapist may aim to raise awareness about this apparent contradiction by saying, "You know, I see you are in need of change, and I gave you a summary of what brings you here. Whatever we call it, it is a way to discuss this, and you react as if you feel you have been overstepped. It's almost too much to take that, and I appreciate that this is important for you to tell me this now. I take this seriously. I also want to tell you that I see you are struggling in your life right now. You are doing all you can to get out of this situation, but you realize you can't escape it alone." The therapist may reformulate Irene's attacking behavior as related to her need for treatment and change. Attacking the therapist is just one means to attain her fundamental motives, though it is highly unusual and negative. If this intervention is done in a timely and authentic way, we may expect the patient to acknowledge her need for treatment at this point, and her attacking behavior may disappear completely.

Transference-Focused Perspective: Bringing Dichotomous Views Into Awareness

From a TFP perspective (Yeomans et al., 2015), working with opposing and dichotomous aspects of the self and experiences of themselves and others is central. Gently bringing those experiences and views of themselves into awareness is crucial. Therapists often do this by focusing on how they are representing themselves and how they are representing others and the vacillation between the two. When Irene said she wanted to be a sex worker, it could be understood as another dichotomous or opposing statement exemplified in the dyad of her fear of other people exposing her sexuality and, at other times, her talking about exposing her sexuality through sex work. The concern that brought her into therapy preexisted; it did not materialize at the therapist's diagnosis. Yet, the therapist's diagnosis may help the patient develop a more nuanced and integrated picture of her need for change.

Dialectical Behavior Perspective: Developing Awareness of Dichotomous Coping States

From a DBT perspective, it is valuable to examine the dichotomous ways in which individuals sometimes present in terms of their emotion regulation. In Irene's case, aspects of her presentation indicate difficulties in communicating and expressing her emotional needs. However, she also portrays herself as someone who is coping well. She exhibits intelligence and drive in her work, almost to the point of workaholism, and appears to have an intolerance for acknowledging any personal shortcomings. This intolerance may be rooted in her belief that she cannot show any weaknesses and holds high expectations for herself, leading her to inhibit, dismiss, or expect herself always to be competent and capable. Growing up in an environment where competence was valued, Irene finds it challenging to reveal any vulnerabilities in her character. While she may manage by concealing her problems, setting high work standards, and working long hours, she becomes dysregulated when her fallibility is brought to her attention.

Despite presenting herself as someone who is coping, Irene is struggling to cope. It is noteworthy that at her age, she relies on her mother's presence during therapy sessions, which can be seen as quite passive. On the one hand, she presents as an intelligent and hardworking professional who maintains a "no problem" attitude, denying the existence of any personality disorders. On the other hand, she allows herself to depend on her mother for support and accompaniment, even at the age of 28. There is a vacillation between the belief "I must be completely capable and competent without any problems" and "I am someone who cannot cope and needs to rely on others, like my mother, to assist me in making appointments." If this pattern persists, it becomes crucial to enhance Irene's awareness of it. When she is in a more competent state, it is important to help her recognize any inhibited, suppressed, dismissed, or disavowed emotional experiences. Conversely, when she is in a more passive and seemingly incapable state, it is important to empower her to become more proactive and build her confidence, capability, and self-efficacy.

Maintaining a Productive Emotion Focus in the Face of Cognitive-Perceptual Disturbances

From our case formulations, it appears that maintaining a productive emotional focus may be important for the work with Irene, as it is for many patients with difficulties in this functional domain. Also, cognitive–perceptual disturbances can be a sequela of dysregulated emotion. While we have a specific quote from Irene's material to anchor this clinical choice point, there are many examples. For example, when Irene described her history of failed occupational experiences, she became angry and defiant, and her thinking became more rigid; her attention narrowly focused on becoming a sex trade worker. When a patient becomes emotionally dysregulated, it can be challenging to tactfully highlight that their thinking is extreme. Building the patient's emotional awareness and regulatory capacity can help develop more realistic thinking. Across all choice points, helping Irene develop a language for her emotions can help her more accurately perceive situations and interrupt extreme and rigid thinking. When working on undoing the transient psychotic state, it can help to identify the precise moment that led to the extreme thinking and the underlying emotions that contributed to the escalated cognitive symptoms and develop a more modulated response.

We agree it is important to recognize that there are often underlying mental states or emotions that relate to the expressed emotions. This is true from mentalization-based therapy, TFP, DBT, and emotion-focused therapy perspectives and probably many others. Often, patients with narcissistic personality disorder respond with hostility and anger when they experience negative evaluations of themselves or fears of vulnerability to getting close and longing for dependence. This pattern is not only observed in patients with pathological narcissism but also various other patients, including Irene. This patient pushes for independence in the face of her dependency needs. Longing for closeness with others or to be taken care of is a strong desire for many that can evoke the anxiety of being mistreated or not looked after in a satisfying way, so people tend to defend against it. Across the various therapies, while there are, in general, diverse terminology and methods, fundamentally, there are many commonalities and overlapping processes.

Building emotion regulation skills should include helping patients differentiate between adaptive and maladaptive emotions. While all emotions contain adaptive and precious information about survival, some emotions, such as Irene's anger when she attacks the therapist, are less immediately informative of and conducive to adaptation and survival (e.g., when she acknowledges that she needs help and suffers greatly). Here, an emotion focus involves differentiating between adaptive and maladaptive primary emotions and secondary or instrumental ones, each requiring different therapist interventions (Greenberg, 2015; Greenberg & Angus, 2003). When Irene exhibits impulsive behaviors, such as making rash decisions or attacking the therapist, one may assume those symptoms are the by-product of her escaping some aversive emotional experience. From a DBT perspective, it may be important to increase her ability to observe, describe, and differentiate the emotional experience. When Irene reacts with an angry outburst, she needs to recognize and distinguish between the primary emotion and the secondary emotional response (e.g., the angry outburst). In other words, if the angry outburst serves as an escape from another underlying aversive emotion that may be intolerable to her, we may want to help her increase her ability to tolerate it. We need to help Irene become aware of what triggers her emotional responses and help her observe, describe, and distinguish primary emotions from secondary emotions. If she can do that, she is less likely to modulate her emotions by relying on behaviors that are impulsive, dysfunctional, or rooted in any kind of escape.

SUMMARY STATEMENT: HOW TO MOVE TOWARD A COHERENT AND REALITY-BASED NARRATIVE

Addressing the functional domain of cognitive–perceptual disturbance in patients with personality disorders can be challenging, but it is central for change. In this chapter, we presented diverse clinical perspectives that may point to a potential mechanism of change. Broadly speaking, the development of a coherent narrative, one that is grounded in logical causal connections and reality and that takes into account the opposing mental states, may be a key change process in recovery. While this global formulation seems logical, research is lacking to support this claim. Currently, there is a lack of research examining whether the development of a coherent and reality-based narrative is predictive of positive outcomes in psychotherapy for personality disorders. In what follows, we summarize the insights gained from our discussion of Irene's case.

Several common methods were recommended to address Irene's cognitive–perceptual distortions and help her develop a more coherent and reality-based sense of herself and others. An important first step with a patient who manifests severe cognitive–perceptual disturbances, including transient psychotic states, begins with an assessment of the severity and scope of the problem. This typically entails conducting a diagnostic assessment. Understanding whether the symptoms are due to an independent psychotic disorder or are related to personality decompensation is critical to managing the patient's symptoms.

When addressing transient psychotic states, it is helpful for the therapist to adopt an open-minded and nonjudgmental stance. It is important for the therapist to remain interested and compassionate toward the patient, especially in response to the discussion of sensitive issues, such as conflicting areas of the narrative and reality. The therapist can express interest in the quasipsychotic processes to deepen their understanding of the patient and to clarify how firmly held the patient's views are.

Transient psychotic states may be surface manifestations of psychopathology that represent avoidance strategies or maneuvers that defend the patient from core vulnerable experiences. Quasipsychotic experiences can arise in response to perceived threats to the patient's sense of self, such as information that is inconceivable or not tolerated by the patient. In Irene's case, we hypothesized that her discussions about her conflict with her father and his threat of withdrawing financial support might be overwhelming for her. Irene appears to engage in a number of strategies to avoid this threat, such as ruminating about being threatened by coworkers. Focusing on the patient's avoidance maneuvers and highlighting the content being avoided and the pain of this situation may be a productive avenue for change when facing cognitive disturbance.

Initially, it is advisable to avoid directly confronting the patient with the absurdness of the content too early on. For example, in the case of Irene, we recommend taking the transient delusional content of the "website" seriously and directly exploring and listening to the patient's concerns about the website. Also, to strengthen the alliance, the therapist should take the content of the cognitive disturbance seriously.

While working with severe cognitive disturbance or dissociation, it is important to help the patient focus on the emotions underlying the transient psychotic content. Some helpful strategies include inviting the patient to observe their emotional state, reflecting the patient's expressed emotions, or empathizing and reflecting the emotions that are not directly expressed but are a core theme underlying the content. For example, in the case of Irene, she expressed thoughts about people posting sensitive and damaging information about her, which reflected an underlying feeling of helplessness, powerlessness, and fear.

When addressing a patient with severe cognitive dysfunction who is struggling to make rational decisions, the therapist should handle opposing content by balancing opposing contents or stances. For example, in the case of Irene, who impulsively claims that she is going to become a sex worker, the therapist can acknowledge the patient's freedom to be in control of her life while simultaneously expressing concerns about the negative consequences of the patient's decision. It is often tricky to navigate these situations because a therapist can come across as attempting to control the patient's life and decisions, and this would likely precipitate a rupture in the therapeutic alliance (see Chapter 9 for navigation of ruptures).

When responding to a patient who exhibits inconsistent and confusing content, it is important to help them integrate their thinking into less extreme, less polarized views and develop a reality-based, coherent narrative. This may be achieved by helping the patient consider new information outside their awareness. In the case of Irene, this may involve increasing her awareness of her desire to be helped and the impact of her critical behavior toward her therapist.

When intervening with a patient who exhibits transient psychotic states, the "loudest" emotions may not necessarily be the most important ones to focus on. The expressed emotions may be secondary to vulnerable primary emotions rooted in painful developmental experiences. Most emotion-focused therapeutic approaches take into account such a view of emotions; this differentiated emotion lens is particularly important for patients with personality disorders.

Some differences in our approach to the case of Irene were evident at the level of specific recommended strategies. The DBT perspective emphasized attention to the here and now, an emotion focus throughout, and skills coaching to increase the patient's awareness of the components of emotional experience, including triggers, bodily sensations, and action urges. A primary aim of DBT is to strengthen the patient's capacity to regulate their emotions, including modulating impulsive actions; helping a patient connect with their intuitive or "wise mind" can inhibit impulsive and irrational behavior. The TFP perspective encouraged grounding the patient in the here-and-now emotional experience but emphasized greater use of interpretation and recognition of fantasies. Finally, the plan analytic approach also recommended a focus on awareness of emotional experience; however, it focused more on the awareness of primary adaptive emotions and identifying and articulating existential needs.

For the integration of dichotomous aspects, TFP offers a lens focusing on dyad representations that can oscillate from one moment to the next within the therapeutic relationship with the current therapist. DBT conceptualizes these dichotomous aspects as the patient's dialectical dilemmas that call for a solution. Clarification-oriented psychotherapy, which partially builds on the model of plan analysis, offers an understanding of two types of opposing action-regulation processes: motive-near and externally focused strategic processes.

The recommended strategies, taken together, may readily be incorporated by therapists who work from an integrative perspective when treating a patient experiencing severe cognitive dysregulation problems. The ongoing clinical challenge remains how to intervene at a particular therapeutic moment or choice point; in line with this discourse, we invoke the adage that several roads lead to Rome (but not necessarily the same roads work for all patients). Finally, our focus on moving a patient from cognitively disturbed thinking into a more coherent and reality-consistent narrative involves different threads that suggest potential mechanisms of change that could be examined in future research.

9

CHALLENGES IN THE THERAPEUTIC RELATIONSHIP AND HOW TO USE THEM PRODUCTIVELY IN PSYCHOTHERAPY

Cultivating a positive relationship in psychotherapy is important but can be challenging when treating individuals with personality disorders; this chapter explores these challenges. We examine how therapists manage counter-therapeutic reactions, observe personal limits, and navigate the formation, ruptures, and repairs in the therapeutic alliance. In this chapter, we review the empirical literature on the relationship between the therapeutic alliance and outcomes in the treatment of personality disorders. We follow by presenting the case of Maria, a woman whose treatment was marked by challenges in the therapeutic relationship.[1] Our case discussion focuses on the relationship challenges, our clinical formulation, and general considerations for structuring therapy. We identify choice points that emerged from our observations. We share theories and clinical opinions to collectively create insight into how the productive use of relationship challenges in therapy may act as a mechanism of change, explaining treatment effects.

---

[1]The case of Maria has been modified to disguise her identity and protect her confidentiality.

https://doi.org/10.1037/0000388-010
Understanding Mechanisms of Change in Psychotherapies for Personality Disorders, by U. Kramer, K. N. Levy, and S. McMain

For us, addressing relationship challenges in treatments for patients with personality disorders is a central task but not anchored in a specific functional domain, as explicated in Chapter 2. This is because we understand relationship challenges as a dyadic phenomenon, which cannot unequivocally be attributed to patient personality functioning or difficulties. Therefore, while also based on a dialogue among the authors and acknowledging the contributions of both patient and therapist to the process, the structure of this chapter is slightly different from the previous five. Specifically, before discussing choice points, we offer a possible therapy structure and a general psychotherapeutic stance for working with the patient. The clinical choice points then focus on the need for further information and clarification, avoiding a rupture in the relationship, and building trust. For each choice point, we offer our combined perspective on therapeutic work on relationship challenges rather than outlining individual approaches. Finally, we end with a synthesized statement to take into account the underlying emotional vulnerability that may be found in a number of functional domains. The focus on emotion is discussed to address these relationship challenges.

RESEARCH ON THE THERAPY RELATIONSHIP IN INDIVIDUALS WITH PERSONALITY DISORDERS

A number of studies have examined relationship challenges in psychotherapy with personality disorders, including poor collaboration between patient and therapist, alliance strains, and the expression of negative affect toward the therapist. We observe that many of these studies are insufficient to provide explicit clinical guidance addressing the complexity of the therapeutic interaction. Consistent with the broader literature, research has revealed that the therapeutic alliance is a reliable predictor of improved outcomes in the treatment of individuals with personality disorders (Flückiger et al., 2018), although more research is needed on this issue. Relative to research on other disorders, the association between the alliance and outcome in those with borderline personality disorder (BPD) is more variable (ranging between a .00 and .79 correlation; Flückiger et al., 2018). It is unclear what the reasons for this large variability are. As an analog to the high variance of the alliance-outcome relationship, researchers have described a rather high intraindividual fluctuation of alliance ratings across psychotherapy in samples where patients presented with a personality disorder (e.g., Hirsh et al., 2012; Kramer et al., 2014). Indeed, session-by-session fluctuations in the quality of the collaboration may represent a challenge for researchers interested in studying the clinically relevant process and clinicians who need effective concepts to address relationship challenges. Collaboration with a patient diagnosed with a personality disorder, particularly BPD, can fluctuate moment-by-moment within a session, requiring a far more complex conceptualization than using the average therapeutic alliance as an indicator. After all, relationship challenges frequently arise at particular moments in psychotherapy and demand immediate resolution.

Given these limitations, it may be preferable to conceptualize the therapeutic relationship in treatments for personality disorders in terms of the moment-by-moment fluctuation of mental states in the collaboration (Levy et al., 2010), repairs of momentary ruptures in the therapeutic alliance (Boritz et al., 2018; Cash et al., 2014; Muran & Eubanks, 2020), appropriate therapist responsiveness (Culina et al., 2022; Kramer, 2021), and other specific relationship descriptors that may explain the development and maintenance of a strong alliance.

Ruptures in the therapeutic alliance and their repair by the common efforts of the patient and therapist may be a particularly fruitful avenue to understanding relationship challenges and how they can be put to productive use in therapy. In a meta-analysis on the impact of specific training in the repair of therapy alliance ruptures by therapists on the patient's outcomes, Eubanks et al. (2018) found that the presence of a personality disorder affected the results as a moderating variable. In other words, it may be less effective to train therapists to resolve alliance ruptures with patients with personality disorders than those without personality disorders (see also Eubanks et al., 2022). It seems clear that such alliance rupture resolution strategies are the most needed for these patients, given the relationship difficulties (i.e., aloofness, dominance, hostility, antagonism) observed in some patients with personality disorders.

In line with these observations, research has shown that the expression of patient hostility influences spontaneous in-session therapist responsiveness for personality disorders. A study by Anderson et al. (2012) found that patients' expressions of hostility in the first session impacted the further process and outcome of psychotherapy. Subtle hostile communication by patients was associated with more patient disclosures and edifications, more therapist interpretations and edifications, and fewer therapist questions and reflections than nonhostile communications. This means that patients process characteristics, such as expression of hostility in session, that affect the course of therapist responsiveness. Of note, the variability observed in correlations between various process characteristics (e.g., the alliance) and outcome may also be due to the influence of the underlying responsiveness effect (Stiles, 2009).

While conceptualizations of responsiveness generally focus on what the therapist uses when they respond to the patient ("being responsive with," e.g., empathy, validation, interpretation, support), less attention is given to what the therapist may be responsive to. The latter may include patient manifestations, such as negative affect, criticism, and a lack of collaboration; thus, they represent the pragmatic challenges therapists face in session. In this context, it may be useful to differentiate between three levels of granularity in what the therapist may be responsive to (Kramer, 2021): They may be responsive to any patient behaviors ("generic": The therapist expresses empathy to all patient manifestations), disorder-specific behaviors ("disorder-specific": The therapist focuses on patient-related disorder-specific processes, such as emotion regulation or mentalizing), or ideographically selected behaviors ("individualized": The therapist uses a case formulation to decide which patient behavior will be complementary and which will not for a particular patient). In a process-outcome analysis on explaining the progression of the therapeutic alliance, it was found that the generic and individualized models predicted the progression of the alliance, and only the individualized conceptualization of therapist responsiveness was related to symptom decrease (Kramer, 2021). More research must consider these dynamics between patients with personality pathology and their therapists, assuming that both interaction partners influence each other on all time scales and, thus, contribute to a potential relationship challenge in psychotherapy.

THE CASE OF MARIA

Maria, a self-identifying woman, is 42 years old, White, heterosexual, and single. She presents to therapy because of a "general dissatisfaction with life." She has a history of self-harming behaviors that currently seem under control, though she has latent suicidal thoughts. Maria meets the criteria for major depression, with marked irritability, feelings of hopelessness and guilt, and low mood, as well as BPD, with identity difficulties, affective instability, marked impulsivity, self-harming behavior and suicidal thoughts, and instability in interpersonal relationships. From our clinical assessment, using the *Diagnostic and Statistical Manual of Mental Disorders* (5th ed., text rev.; American Psychiatric Association, 2022) alternative model five trait domains, Maria scored high on affective instability, disinhibition, and antagonism and average on detachment and psychoticism.

Maria has a long history of abusive intimate relationships dating back to young adulthood. Maria was an only child whose parents separated when she was 7 years old, after which she was raised by her mother and only saw her father occasionally. Maria described her father as "impulsive" and an alcoholic;

she described her mother as passive, with moments of expressed hostility. She denied any experiences of physical or sexual abuse in her childhood but always felt "different" and "somewhat excluded" from her peers. When she began the current treatment, she had been in a 6-year-long intimate relationship with a man she portrayed as "dormant" and "sleepy." She was also engaged in an affair with her boss. Maria is a trained and certified nurse. After working several years as a nurse with relative success but overall dissatisfaction with the hospital staff she worked with, Maria abruptly decided to quit her job and train as an herbal therapist. When therapy began, Maria had been working at a private practice as an herbal therapist for 2 years. Although she was excited about becoming an herbal therapist, overall, Maria feels fundamentally unhappy and describes her life as "an unhappy shithole."

Maria had been in psychoanalysis for 10 years. She angrily declared that this experience "made things worse." She loudly declared, "Before entering psychoanalysis, I had a life. Now, I am destroyed, and I am deep in debt." Although it appeared that Maria was not improving from psychoanalysis and was continuing to have problems, her description of her life was rosy before starting psychoanalysis. The amount of deterioration that occurred subsequently was discordant to how she described her functioning at the beginning of her analysis. In addition, although Maria had been unhappy with her therapy and ambivalent about it for some time, she terminated treatment precipitously and unilaterally without discussing it with her therapist. Subsequently, she experienced a precipitous increase in suicidal thoughts, which she voiced to others as threats. Three months later, her distress and suicidal urges motivated her to pursue another treatment with her current psychotherapist.

In her first session, Maria appeared somewhat detached as she recounted several aspects of her history. Her affect appeared well-regulated as she answered questions in a straightforward and seemingly informative manner. On the one hand, her responses struck the therapist as similar to a compliant student answering a teacher's questions. On the other hand, it felt to the therapist that she was subtly seeking reassurance from them. Although somewhat dominant in her manner and lacking in warmth in her nonverbal behavior, she was a likable person.

During the second session, Maria arrived with a suitcase and a large bag; she commented that she had slept at her boss's house as part of their affair and came directly to the session. When the therapist explored her motivation for further treatment since her termination of therapy with her psychoanalyst, Maria paused and then, with contempt, stated that her psychoanalyst had only made things worse. She also expressed hostility and contempt toward the therapist and made a special point of indicating that she is a therapist herself and knows what she needs. She then demanded antidepressants, saying, "I need a good and strong therapy, not your questions." The second session is explored in more detail when discussing clinical choice points later in this chapter.

This information was a stimulus for a discussion about how to conceptualize Maria's case from our three perspectives. The case formulations are compared with regard to similarities and differences. We put forward a treatment frame for Maria's case and developed several options for intervening, with a focus on the relationship challenge. We conclude by summarizing general principles that may help address relationship challenges, such as the one found in Maria's case.

CASE FORMULATION: UNDERSTANDING RELATIONSHIP CHALLENGES AND DYNAMICS WITHIN THE THERAPEUTIC CONTEXT

Case formulation is the basis for providing meaning from complex and often ambiguous information. It may be particularly relevant for understanding relationship aspects and offers a coherent framework for intervention. We begin by considering how to conceptualize Maria's relationship problems and how they may manifest in the therapy hour. Because a nuanced understanding of the relationship challenges and dynamics is important, this section on case formulation is particularly detailed.

Maria appeared angry about previous treatments. Her choice of words—that it was a "really bad therapy" that left her "destroyed"—are strong statements. Although they are possibly true and consistent with Maria's phenomenological experience, they may be overstated. One hypothesis is that Maria believes the current therapist would not understand the impact the earlier therapy had on her without the use of such strong words. There was also a defensive and angry quality to her narrative, and she expressed anger toward the therapist.

Transference-Focused Formulation: Understanding the Therapeutic Relationship Via Past Relationships

From a transference-focused psychodynamic model, the therapist examined how the patient experiences others, such as the previous therapist, boss, and coworkers. Understanding Maria's relationships with others may help the therapist anticipate how she might experience the therapist. She may perceive the current therapist as similar to how she described her previous therapist. Maria's comments about how all therapy is about conning people, making them worse, and having ulterior motives may be understood from an object relation dyad theoretical lens, though it is also possible that this particular dynamic is not part of a specific object relation dyad.

From this perspective, it would be assumed that Maria would question the therapist's motives and whether this therapy is helpful. Maria makes it difficult to understand her by not sharing openly. Her attitude is, in part, one of "you should know" and "I shouldn't have to tell you." Although, at one level, we might understand that Maria has experienced many people as unhelpful and having malevolent motives, this stance makes it difficult for the therapist to understand and help her. From a transference-focused perspective, Maria's stance toward the therapist presents an opening for exploring her expectations and the dynamics underlying them.

From a transference-focused psychotherapy (TFP) viewpoint, focusing on object relation dyads involves paying attention to the person's representation of themselves and others. These representations are interrelated, such that whenever the person has a representation of themselves, they also have a representation of the other, and vice versa. For example, if one feels competent and worthy of love, one sees that other people might view them that way as well. Conversely, if one views others as perpetrators and aggressors, one might see oneself as somebody who has been a victim of other people's control. From a TFP perspective, we would expect Maria's representations of herself to vacillate or "flip" with her representation of others. The central idea here is that there are two sides to a representation.

Specifically, Maria sees people as mean-spirited, unhelpful, and attacking, almost as if "they say they are going to, but they are not going to help you." Maria may not only experience other people that way but also experience herself that way. Evidence for the latter is seen when she sits quietly and does not say much. In these moments, she is withholding and not completely forthcoming. In some ways, she withholds information when she thinks other people are withholding information from her.

From a TFP perspective, like other perspectives, it is assumed that people's behavior represents the best they can do, given their experiences and circumstances, and that these behaviors may work in certain situations but often in limited ways. But as in dialectical behavior therapy (DBT), it is important to understand that although there may be some value in the behavior, there are other consequences that are undesirable to the patient, as they themselves often articulate. In addition, we assume Maria could present as a "good girl," not saying anything and not disrupting things, but it also appears that she can say a lot of nasty things about her boyfriend, her work, and the therapist. So, one can assume there is aggression there, too.

At times, Maria is likely to experience herself one way and, at other times, quite differently, but she may not be aware of these disparate representations of herself. Therefore, she cannot get a consistent image of herself or her direction, which may contribute to the identity problems described earlier. Either she is withdrawing (often in a hostile manner) and thus not participating, or she is involved, albeit erratically and contemptuous of the other. The goal of therapy is to gently make her aware of these despaired aspects of her experience so she can become more flexible and have a more integrated experience of herself. Even saying, "I'm scared to tell my therapist this, but I think I'm going to try because if I don't tell them, how are they going to know how I feel?" may be an opening to a corrective emotional experience within psychotherapy.

In conclusion, the TFP formulation of Maria's relationship challenge may focus on her contradictory inner experiences in her relationships with others, either being a "good girl," submissive and self-effacing, or being "nasty" and aggressive. The therapeutic relationship with this therapist becomes the arena where the patient's inner inconsistencies are played out. The role of the therapist is to notice these changes, or "flips," moment by moment, and the challenge will become to contain these fluctuations and move toward fostering a broader sense of self.

Dialectical Behavior Formulation: Biological and Environmental Causes of Relationship Problems

From a DBT perspective, Maria's therapist believed that her struggles stem from an inability to regulate her emotions effectively. This deficit likely developed due to inherent emotional vulnerability and a history of invalidating experiences. The therapist identified Maria's emotional regulation as the root cause behind her problematic behaviors, such as anger outbursts, suicidal thoughts, and unsatisfying relationship dynamics. A central theme that emerged is Maria's dissatisfaction with others and her perception that they have failed to recognize and respond to her needs. Maria views herself as weak and powerless, which understandably leads to frustration and misery.

Viewed through a DBT lens, Maria's behaviors can be understood and justified considering her biology and upbringing. Her family history suggests the presence of genetic factors contributing to her difficulties with emotion regulation. Maria reported that her father was impulsive and had substance abuse issues, while her mother was passive and nonassertive. Even without a biological predisposition, her challenges in modulating intense emotions and effectively communicating her needs may have arisen from her learning environment. She described growing up in an emotionally volatile household with an alcoholic father, where speaking up and asserting herself may not have been safe. Her mother served as a role model for a nonassertive interpersonal style. Suppressing her thoughts and feelings might have helped Maria feel secure and maintain a connection with her parents. However, this lack of nurturance, support, and validation likely hindered her ability to accept and tolerate painful emotions. Consequently, she may have learned to distrust and invalidate her experiences, making it difficult for her to identify her needs.

This difficulty in asserting herself is evident in her description of her previous therapist relationship. Despite feeling dissatisfied, Maria did not voice her concerns or take any action. She may have been unaware of her emotional needs in that relationship, or expressing them might have felt risky. Her pattern of neglecting her needs became apparent through her compliant and submissive behavior with her therapist. Continuously inhibiting and dismissing her needs with others could contribute to her growing resentment and frustration. These negative emotions frequently arise in her relationships, with Maria feeling taken advantage of due to the belief that she is not being seen or considered. The unsatisfying relationships Maria described, likely stemming from earlier invalidating experiences, may also manifest in her relationship with the therapist.

In conclusion, from a DBT perspective, issues within the therapeutic relationship can arise from Maria's emotional vulnerability and her past experiences with significant individuals. It appears challenging for Maria to express her needs and have them met. The therapist's task, therefore, is to address the underlying emotional vulnerability while being attentive to the repetitive patterns in Maria's relationship experiences, including the therapeutic one.

Plan Analysis Formulation: Contextualizing Relationship Problems Within Possible Therapist Behaviors

From a plan analysis perspective, it may be important to conceptualize these difficult, at times hostile, interaction situations in terms of what sort of therapist behaviors are (a) conducive to even more relationship challenges or (b) more functional in terms of a corrective relationship experience for Maria. To answer this question, it may be good to take a step back and reflect on the behaviors Maria is engaging in and her experiences in the therapy hour. She is hostile to the therapist, expressing contempt and defying their role as a psychotherapist who could be a resource for her ("I need a good and strong treatment, not your questions"). These behaviors, while potentially difficult for the therapist, may indicate how she usually interacts with meaningful people in her life, expresses vulnerability, or expresses when she is in need. From a plan analysis case formulation perspective (Caspar, 2019, 2022), it may be important to ask what purpose(s) these behaviors and experiences serve. Perhaps Maria expresses hostility to present as a "difficult" patient, or she wants to ensure the current therapist knows she already had certain (in her sense, failed) psychotherapy experiences.

This interpersonal presentation may serve a higher plan to make sure the therapist is willing to give their best and go "the extra mile." Underlying this plan may be a strong sense of being unseen and hurt in interpersonal relationships while at the same time expecting that she may be hurt again in the current therapeutic relationship. While the patient is unaware of this process, it may help us understand which interpersonal behaviors the therapist should adopt in a complementary fashion (by focusing on the underlying motive) to create optimal conditions for Maria to have a corrective relationship experience in this therapy. Here, the therapist could give specific relationship messages (as discussed later) to Maria on how difficult it must be for her and, by the same means, express that they are particularly interested in the extraordinary difficulties she has in managing her life (resulting in a sense of "being stuck" and a life that is "nonexistent"), despite all the competencies the patient seems to have (e.g., as an herbal therapist with a diploma).

There is also material suggesting some internal contradictions within the patient; however, it may be too early at Session 2 to use this information to keep the emotional intensity at an optimal level. For example, it seems astonishing to observe the intensity of Maria's difficulties, knowing she is working as a therapist herself and is therefore exposed to difficult interactions daily. Treatment would involve the therapist offering motive-oriented interventions that aim at "seeing" or recognizing the underlying motives or motivations for "getting better" (i.e., healing), coming to the session, expressing the difficulties to a therapist (time and again), and aiming at formulating a treatment focus. The case formulation will inform the therapist on what to do in the relationship: Understand what is going on and what is needed from the therapist to create the conditions for possible relationship healing in terms of a corrective emotional experience.

In conclusion, from a plan analytic case formulation perspective, Maria's challenges in the therapeutic relationship appear to serve interpersonal functions that may involve sending a message to the therapist that they need to commit fully to therapy or that some kind of mobilizing treatment may be needed. Here, the challenge is understood as meeting the patient on the level of the underlying motives rather than on the level of responding directly to the constraining interaction behaviors Maria is engaged in to create a new and corrective relationship experience.

Toward a Common Formulation

We observe that our three perspectives of case formulation largely overlap. We understand Maria as a patient who is highly conflictual and momentarily hostile to others and as someone who also presents with a number of strengths and resources (e.g., being able to deal with difficult patients herself). Maria puts the current therapist in a highly uncomfortable and challenging situation by criticizing the therapist and expressing contempt and hostility. We partially disagree when explaining what is driving the expression of hostility, as shown in these excerpts. A transference-focused lens assumes a constant readiness to flip (a moment-by-moment fluctuation of affective-relational states involving opposites of an object relation dyad) between different states in the here and now. A dialectical behavior lens assumes that emotional vulnerability interacts with Maria's difficulty expressing her needs due to her learned experience. A plan analytic lens assumes that hostile behavior may be underpinned by interpersonal motives, such as signaling to the therapist that they should go "the extra mile" in the context of the present therapy. While different formulations will lead to different intervention options, as discussed later, Maria's problematic interaction behavior calls for fostering a new relationship experience in the here and now, which may be called, according to certain therapy models, "corrective."

CHOICE POINTS AND OPPORTUNITIES FOR CHANGE

In this section, we discuss how we can intervene effectively and use specific therapy moments as opportunities for change, according to what we know from our case formulations of Maria's situation and the research presented in the chapter's introduction. We start by discussing our different contributions to the general choice points on the structure of therapy and the therapist's stance on the relationship challenge posed by Maria's case and move forward by offering insights on how to address some of the specific choice points that have manifested in the excerpts. We suggest focusing on navigating at the edge of an alliance rupture toward building trust.

What Kind of Therapy Structure Is Needed?

Irrespective of whether Maria's interpersonal behaviors are understood in terms of relationship dyads, difficulties in emotion regulation, or context-activated plans and behavior underlying motives, we observe that Maria expresses discontent, even contempt, toward the therapist in these early therapy sessions. While the origin of this expression may be attributable to early-life dynamics of relational misattunement and neglect by attachment figures, the relationship challenge is in the present, and the therapist is called to intervene in a context marked by a certain pressure. Having Maria commit to this treatment within a context of sufficient trust and at least a somewhat positive therapeutic relationship is the therapist's current overarching task in these early therapy sessions. Developing a "therapy frame" as part of the collaboration and the therapeutic alliance is an essential component that increases Maria's commitment to therapy. For example, directly discussing the financial aspects of the therapy should happen as early as possible, particularly because Maria voiced concern about the finances of her previous therapy experiences. This may decrease the probability of misunderstanding and contribute to a clear frame and a trusting, transparent relationship. Also, having an agenda and structure may help to get things done in the session, although not all therapists may feel the need for such structure during the session. While session structure may decrease the spontaneous expression of the patient during the session, it may also inhibit some of Maria's negative feelings and instill hope for change. It is an open question whether those negative feelings should be fully expressed at this point (see the later discussion on emotion focus).

With the development of the therapy frame in mind, there are limits to such an expression early on in treatment because it may undermine the development of the collaboration, trust, and focus of the therapeutic work. The importance of engaging well with patients such as Maria should not be underestimated. One study showed that the quality of the treatment frame positively affects outcome and negatively affects dropout (in the sense of fewer early terminations; Yeomans et al., 1994). Importantly, addressing the treatment frame works when the therapist avoids imposing anything on the patient; the construction of the frame is, again, collaborative.

Which Therapist Stance Is Useful in Facing Relationship Challenges?

Fundamentally, the therapist should aim to be present and fully respectful when facing Maria's experience. The therapist should aim to work hard to hear what Maria has to say and should be attentive if they think the patient is not experiencing them that way. Among the most important factors is that Maria feels she has no control over the situation or interaction. In the situation with her current therapist, she feels she has no control and is trying to assert her control. When she gets upset, it may be good for the therapist to tolerate her anger, contain it, and tolerate what is talked about. Sometimes it is helpful to use what are called, in the context of psychodynamic psychotherapies, "therapist-centered techniques" when the patient challenges the relationship by saying, "You're a rotten therapist. You don't know what you're doing." It is assumed the therapist does not necessarily believe that about themselves while recognizing they are not the best therapist in the country either. This may represent a distortion, but it is the patient's legitimate experience of the therapist. To avoid reinforcing the distortion, the therapist may say, "Yeah, I am a rotten therapist. I don't know what I'm doing," but by doing so, it is possible for the patient to feel invalidated. So, as an alternative, they can say, "I can imagine how difficult it would be to come to therapy and sit with somebody who you think doesn't know what they're doing." In this case, the therapist is not admitting that they do not know what they are doing but formulates it by taking the patient's perspective.

This therapist-centered technique from psychodynamic psychotherapy may be similar to other relationship interventions, such as validation in DBT, in which the therapist also takes the patient's perspective. However, therapist-centered interventions are usually more advantageous when the therapist is in an interpersonally challenging situation, such as in Maria's case. Alternatively, Maria's expression about the "rotten" therapist may also allow her to test the therapist's resilience in handling tough interaction moments and thus allow her, eventually, and if the therapist focuses on her central motive, to develop more trust in the therapeutic relationship.

We agree that it is important for the therapist to be honest and transparent with Maria. We think the first thing the therapist should say to Maria as soon as she sits down is, "I know a little bit about what brings you here from talking to Dr. Bolva [Maria's previous therapist] and from reading the notes [or from a phone call, an email, or another method of communication with Maria], but it would be useful for me to hear, in your own words, what it is that you are hoping to get out of this and what brings you here. How do you understand the nature of your difficulties? What are you hoping to get out of the treatment? How are things for you right now?" The patient might then say, "I want help with my relationship," or "Although I am with my boyfriend, I am having an affair, but I am happy with that." Alternatively, the therapist could ask, "What do you want my help with?" With this question, the therapist takes an interpersonally submissive stance and empowers Maria by giving her control of therapy. The benefit of doing so is that it can help increase a sense of collaboration and engagement.

Therapists need to acknowledge their contribution to a relationship challenge. It is possible that the therapist is not focusing enough on the therapeutic relationship in the here and now, possibly interfering slightly with the development of the patient's trust in the early moments of therapy and contributing to the relationship challenge. For example, one could wonder what the purpose is of Maria being so dominant with this therapist. What is the purpose of her asking for a particularly effective treatment, and what is the purpose of her stating that she is a therapist as well? These behaviors all have motivational underpinnings that are still unclear but may be tentatively accessible by doing a case formulation (see our earlier integrative attempt at a formulation). Is she engaging in these behaviors to ensure the therapist pays particular attention to her as someone who is competent? Or do they serve another purpose? For example, they may make sure that others never bring her down or criticize her. Using this formulation will help provide a direction for the therapist to know how to intervene at the relationship level, which operates mostly using nonverbal and paraverbal means of expression.

Importantly, despite the therapist's intention to not try to put Maria down, we must acknowledge that she might still feel this way. This may focus on the patient's representation or experience of the event rather than the actual event. For example, if Maria expresses annoyance in response to the therapist's question, "Can you say more about that?" the therapist's answer may be, "I noticed—and tell me if I don't get this right—that when I asked you to say more about what you were talking about, you were annoyed with me. Maybe just slightly, but I think it was enough that it is worth examining." Maria may say, "Yeah, I think I was annoyed." The therapist may say, "Well, do you have any thoughts about what might have been going on?" to which the patient may respond, "Well, I think when you said, 'Can you say more about that?' it seemed you didn't believe what I was saying." Of course, this is not what the therapist meant when they asked the initial question, and the therapist may say, "That is important because I wonder what your thoughts are about it. From my perspective, I was asking because I wanted to hear more about your experience, not that I did not believe your experience." The intention would be to understand Maria's momentary experience better rather than accusing her of lying or assuming certain intentions behind her behavior.

The general therapeutic stance most likely to address Maria's relationship challenge is trying to understand her experience in the here and now, marked by the therapist being honest, transparent, direct, and open to Maria's criticism and questioning the necessity of therapy. This will give Maria the sense of control she may need as she enters this therapeutic relationship.

"I Was Destroyed": The Need for Clarification and More Information

The following is an excerpt from Session 2:

> I did 10 years of therapy, and I am a therapist myself. I know something about therapy, let me tell you. It is just a bad place where weak people are taken advantage of. I was naive. I thought I received help, but instead, I was destroyed.

While the case formulations revealed hypotheses about what we observe and what we know about this patient, there is a need to have additional information, which may be accomplished by doing more assessments and offering clarification. It is important to note that clarification not only increases knowledge on a topic but also offers the patient a chance to dig deeper, inviting them to elaborate and clarify more. Maria said she had undergone long-term psychoanalysis, but we do not know why. Maria said she was fine but then was "destroyed" after 10 years of psychoanalysis. The question is why she went to analysis in the first place. What was the concern that brought her to analysis, and how did the situation get to this point? We learned that she is having an affair and is open about it in a way that might end her relationship with her boyfriend and her job. Again, it would be helpful to understand how Maria relates to her current therapist. We do not know what Maria means when she mentions being "destroyed." The therapist should clarify what she means by "destroyed" by asking her to say more about it. The therapist should be careful with the wording to avoid sounding challenging, confronting, invalidating, or interrogative. They should not assume they know what the patient means by "destroyed" in this instance; more detail and context are needed to understand her experience more fully. Given the lack of trust she is experiencing, there may not be a lot of room to challenge this patient, so one might gently remark, "When you say 'destroyed,' can you tell me what that looked like?"

More detailed information on the context of seeking treatment will most likely help this therapist develop more empathy for the patient's current situation. Therefore, clarifying and seeking more information may be helpful, to some extent, to indirectly address the relationship challenge posed by Maria.

"No One Takes Me Seriously": How Can the Therapist Navigate Looming Alliance Ruptures?

The following is a dialogue between the therapist and Maria from Session 2:

THERAPIST: I see this is really painful for you, all this. What's most painful for you right now?

MARIA: Everything together. [*Pauses, sniffs*] I need antidepressants. Can you give me a prescription? I really need it. I thought of suicide a few weeks ago, but no one takes me seriously.

THERAPIST: What do you mean when you say, "No one takes me seriously"?

MARIA: No one. I requested antidepressants from my psychoanalyst, but she did not want to give me any. She thought I was fine. [*Shouts*]

What a professional fault she is! [*Pauses*] So I went to see a family doctor. I looked him up on the internet. What a disaster! How can such a guy be a medical doctor? Awful decorations in the office too. [*Expresses contempt*] Fortunately, I was in there only for 2 minutes. I could not stand him.

THERAPIST: Mm-hmm.

MARIA: The medication did not work. So, I decided to stop them after a few weeks, and I did not go back to the family doctor. They made me dizzy. So, I had just the side effects but no effect. I am a herbal therapist, and I know that medication is not going to work. I knew it from the start.

THERAPIST: What do you mean with . . .

MARIA: I knew no one could help me—at least not this family doctor. My life is nonexistent.

THERAPIST: Yes, you say you need something else . . .

MARIA: And I have to say that the way you ask questions shows me that you don't understand anything. [*Expresses contempt again*] I doubt you can really help me. I am a therapist myself—herbal therapist with a diploma. I know what I need, so I am telling you. I am in such bad shape now that I need antidepressants. And I need a good and strong treatment, not your questions. [*Looks at therapist defiantly*]

A therapist-centered technique, as discussed previously, may have further implications for the level of the therapeutic relationship. It becomes clear that the therapeutic relationship is at stake in these hostile interactions, and a potential alliance rupture or therapy rupture looms large. Some relationship management, building up trust, and a solid basis of collaboration are needed. At the same time, working with the material presented is also an opportunity to foster deeper change and involves seeing the therapeutic relationship itself as a curative element to foster change in this patient.

For example, the patient may say something about how difficult it is to come to therapy and sit with somebody they think is incapable, and a discussion may start from there. The therapist holds the patient's perspective, which is not the same as validating by reinforcing it but rather validating the underlying emotional difficulty. The therapist might say, "What would it be like to be with a therapist that made you feel like this." Or, focusing on the here and now, they might say, "It must be hard for you to say that right now."

In general, to navigate the hostility and address alliance ruptures, any move by the patient toward assertive behavior in the current relationship will be important to reinforce. In this case, it may be important to validate what makes sense about Maria's perspective. For example, the therapist may acknowledge how Maria perceives the therapist's behavior, stating, "I am coming across to you right now as critical" (if that is how she sees the therapist).

The therapist should not shy away from taking responsibility for their contribution to the relationship challenge, which may contribute from certain theoretical viewpoints to fostering a corrective relational experience. For example, if the therapist acknowledges, "I came across as sounding critical," it is important to note that the therapist is not saying the patient said they were intentionally critical but that it may have been how the therapist's comment came across to her. In addition to building an alliance, it would be helpful for Maria to focus on taking any small steps toward asserting herself and taking control (and not being passive). In other words, helping her take responsibility for making choices and encouraging her to take direction would be helpful. Importantly, the therapist assumes, or owns, their contribution to the therapeutic rupture in the alliance or the challenging relationship situation (here, the hostility expressed by the patient).

As a more general choice point but related to addressing the looming rupture, it may be good to weave in more validation throughout the session. Rather than asking a lot of questions, it may be helpful for the therapist to engage less in assessment (which may seem somewhat contrary to the section on clarification earlier) and instead focus on communicating what the therapist is hearing from her. The therapist expresses that there is value in what the patient is saying and conveys that they want to understand her. The therapist's stance should be focused less on direct inquiry and more on the use of understanding the patient's experience through empathic reflection. Here, it is important to attend to both what is being said and what is not being said.

Throughout the session, it may be advisable for the therapist to focus on helping the patient reflect on her thoughts and feelings and supporting her in articulating her needs. The therapist should strive to understand the patient's perspective of the problem and what is bothering her. In these first sessions, it is important to reflect on identifying what is important to the patient and what is in her life. In other words, where does she want to go, what does she value, what is missing in her life, and what is getting in the way of her needs may be leading questions to ask. This would be a way of beginning to clarify the focus of therapy. Rather than the therapist making assumptions about what the patient wants and what she wants from therapy, the therapist wants to help her explicate these goals herself.

In the context of the first sessions, we agree it seems premature to discuss potential problems in the therapy relationship directly. It may be too emotionally charged a conversation with someone who has difficulty asserting her needs with others. Instead, it may be helpful to convey understanding by offering a validating response, such as, "How frustrating it would be to try to get help and not feel like you got the support that you wanted." Again, navigating a specific choice point like this may involve a therapist-centered intervention of the negative affect expressed by the patient.

"I Doubt You Can Help Me": Building Trust in the Therapy Relationship

At Session 2 of the treatment, Maria discussed her affair with her boss and her previous therapy experience in psychoanalysis. On inquiry, she provided a negative picture of the previous therapist and expressed contempt. In the same vein, Maria expressed contempt and hostility to the current therapist by saying, "I doubt you can help me. You know, I am a therapist myself, and I know how it works. Also, I know I need a good and strong therapy, not your questions." At this juncture, a response by her psychotherapist may not be challenging in any way but accepting in the moment: "I appreciate you reminding me that you have expertise here too." It is a response acknowledging that the patient has a perspective the therapist can choose to validate. One might argue that it is interesting that the patient felt she had to remind the therapist of her expertise.

Given this context, there is some agreement among us that the therapist in the vignette is moving somewhat fast by asking a lot of questions (reflected by the patient's statement, "not your questions"), which raises the question of whether the pace of intervention is adequate. While it is good to challenge this patient at one point, it seems the present moment is not the right time. Despite this observation, this therapist offers interventions at a moderately productive but improvable pace. We could imagine that the therapist could also just sit back and listen to the patient's expressed hostility, which is not what is happening. This therapist intervenes regularly and makes statements, thus marking their presence in the therapy relationship. For the patient, to hear that somebody is there and responsive to her may be helpful for her building of trust: the therapist sends an implicit message here that they are attentive and not moving out of the interaction, despite the difficulty it presents. More of this is needed in this case. Proceeding while there is hostility in the room is like sending an implicit relationship message to Maria: "You cannot overcome me with your hostile behavior. I am still here for you." This may go a long way in constructing the collaboration.

In some cases, showing that the therapist understands the patient shows that someone in this universe can understand her experience. This could help Maria feel like there is somebody she may trust in the future.

In these first sessions, it may be important to explore Maria's present struggle and what changes she seeks. For example, the therapist could say, "It sounds so frustrating feeling unsupported by others. I'm wondering if you want my help figuring out ways to develop more satisfying relationships with others?" By stating this as a direct question, the therapist is trying to make the treatment goals explicit.

Navigating a potential alliance rupture involves the therapist being active, being appropriately responsive to the patient's experience in the here and now, and understanding and regulating the therapist's inner experiences as potential countertransferential reactions, as well as their emotions and action tendencies. Openly owning their part in the rupture while adapting the intervention pace to the patient may be central for patients with personality pathology and foster the essential development of trust.

Later in the same session (Session 2), Maria started to cry and said, "This is not a life!" This expression may indicate that she is about to develop more trust in the therapeutic relationship because her statement may indicate that she is opening up to the therapist as a potentially helpful witness to her innermost suffering and a promoter of helping her get a life.

"I Would Fall Apart if I Have to Live Alone": What Should the Therapist Focus On?

The following is dialogue between Maria and the therapist from Session 15:

MARIA: [*Sighs*] It's just that I am so much afraid of not being able to function anymore. It would drive me crazy to be all on my own. I hate my boyfriend. I mean, really, I can't look into his eyes anymore, but at the same time, I am sure that I would fall apart if I have to live alone.

THERAPIST: [*Pauses*] Mm-hmm, so there is this fear of falling apart . . .

MARIA: Mm-hmm. It freaks me out. So I'd rather sleep with my boss, and I have a good sex life like this. Somehow it works for me.

Maria's emotional vulnerability described in our synthesized formulation may lead the therapist to focus on Maria's emotional experience in one or the other way, even in early therapy sessions, which may help address current relationship challenges and contribute to the development of trust in this therapeutic relationship. In the earlier example, the therapist may inquire, "You say 'I would fall apart.' I wonder what this means to you and what you fear when you imagine being alone." Such a focus on the underlying emotional experience may be a different route to further fostering trust in the therapeutic relationship and specifically in the therapist as a witness of her emotional expression and as someone who potentially can propose help and promote further change.

In Session 2, when Maria started to cry and said, "This is not a life," the therapist leaned in empathically, saying, "I see this is really painful for you." Then the therapist attempted to deepen this focus on emotion by inquiring about what may be the most painful in the moment. Maria seemed to protect herself from letting this question unsettle her by saying, "Everything," and insisting that she needed medication, thus diverting the therapist's offer to deepen the emotional experience in the moment. This reaction has been reported in the literature on emotion-focused work with particularly fragile self-organizations—for example, patients with BPD (Pos & Paolone, 2019). When focusing on the patient's emotional experience, therapists will need to give patients with personality pathology more time and provide more elaboration. It is as if patients' overused interpersonal strategies (i.e., their maladaptive interpersonal patterns characteristic of personality disorders; see Chapter 5) intervene at this point and block their access to productive emotional processing. Nevertheless, as early as Session 2 with Maria, the therapist should establish some focus on emotion because this may be useful later in the process, becoming productive (as demonstrated for Maria in Session 15) and contributing to preventing or resolving a relationship challenge. We advise offering any of these interventions (at least one) in the first therapy sessions. Even if the patient does not follow or make immediate use of the intervention, it may be advisable to let them know where the treatment may go and how therapy may work, offering a feeling of what therapy may be like. Focusing on emotional experiences in the here and now has a relationship-building function and may provide Maria with one dimension she may take with her as she leaves the second therapy session: trust in the therapist, which may be seen later in treatment.

It seems that Maria is quickly emotionally activated and then blocks off her emotion, resulting in fluctuating affective states contributing to the relationship challenge (by the expressed emotional negativity addressed by the therapist). At this point, the therapist may say, "It seems like this particular experience [of saying that her life is nonexistent] affects you profoundly. Can you describe your experience right now?" Such an intervention may help Maria be more grounded in the current moment. This can focus on any expressed frustration or positive experience in the here and now. The therapist may want to offer to go as deep as possible into this experience, which may involve how the patient experiences the therapist in the here and now, but not necessarily. Early in therapy, such an intervention focusing on the patient's emotional experience of the therapist would be too difficult for a patient like Maria to process. Another way to start focusing on the emotional experience within the therapeutic relationship may be to ask, "What is it like for you sharing all of this?" which may evolve into "What is it like for you to share all this with me?" This would then open the door to elaborate on the experience with the current therapist and mark the importance of the emotional experience in the therapy room.

If there is evidence that something is going on emotionally, a transference-focused viewpoint would adopt a specific approach consistent with the previous one to foster collaboration. For example, when the therapist gives a patient feedback about their diagnosis, they may say, "Does what I'm saying resonate with you? Does it make sense?" If the patient says yes, the therapist may add, "I am not sure of this, so you can tell me if I have it wrong, but when I hear you say yes the way you just did, almost with a sigh, I wonder if there is a part of you that believes what I am saying, and that is the part that is saying 'yes.' But there is another part of you that may have some doubts about what I am saying, and that is the part that says it tentatively, and I am wondering what all this is like for you right now." It is important to be explicit about the therapist's formulation.

SUMMARY STATEMENT: HOW TO USE CHALLENGES IN THE THERAPEUTIC RELATIONSHIP

Relationship challenges are the bedrock of treatments for patients presenting with personality pathology (and beyond). These challenges often present as moment-by-moment fluctuating expressions of negative affect, direct interpersonal attack or hostility (e.g., the case of Maria), or submissive-hostile withdrawal from collaboration. These challenges may be understood using a variety of lenses of formulation, which imply different intervention options.

Maria presented a multifaceted challenge to the therapeutic relationship, one that we tend to see in highly impaired patients with personality pathology. It seems important to develop a fine ear to listen to Maria's words and be ready to carefully observe her in-session (nonverbal and paraverbal) behavior (e.g., the shakiness in her voice at a certain moment) while at the same time elaborating a grounded explanation of why she may be experiencing reality the way she does. Her words (e.g., implying psychotherapy is destroying her self) may sometimes be understood as distorted overstatements and, at other times, as an expression of an underlying and unexpressed deep interpersonal hurt related to her attachment figures. Her way of presenting herself in the therapeutic relationship may be the repeated pattern understood in the context of specific object relation dyads, her learned incapacity of connecting with her innermost needs, or an unusual way to present as a particularly difficult patient, constraining interaction partners to engage strongly with her. Such a self-presentation is only meaningful as the backdrop of a probably neglectful or traumatic interpersonal experience with her attachment figures, who were described as unable to attend to Maria's need for assertion. She developed (problematic) interpersonal strategies to either "shut" her mouth or present as hostile.

Psychotherapy research has offered systematic insights into relationship variables in therapy; these variables were demonstrated as being most important for effective therapy across diagnoses. While treatments for many psychological disorders have been studied, it may be challenging to take into account the moment-by-moment fluctuations of mental or interpersonal states of patients with personality disorders, particularly BPD. In Maria's case, we observed them as momentary expressed hostility (sometimes in the form of nonverbal contempt). Clearly, administering a postsession questionnaire on the overall quality of the collaboration will inform us about the general thread of collaboration but will miss the subtle intraperson fluctuations: (mini-) ruptures and repairs within the therapeutic relationship. We think that work on fluctuation in in-session emotions could be the future of psychotherapy research to inform a mechanisms-based clinical practice understanding and address relationship challenges.

In Maria's case, there are a few best-practice interventions related to specific choice points that we agree on and some with which we partially disagree. Validating Maria's momentary experience and conveying that the therapist understands her in this situation will ultimately be helpful to Maria. We may also consider that "validating" may feel less validating to her when used on any patient behavior. When facing Maria's hostility, the therapist may use affirmative statements (rather than questions) to make sure Maria gets the sense that someone is seeing her, which may contribute to a change in the relationship experience. Clarification and seeking more information will provide more details the therapist can empathize with.

We agree that, at this early stage of therapy, when facing these relationship challenges, the central therapeutic task is to build an affective bond. Certain therapy models may understand this process as a corrective relationship experience. There are various strategies for how this may be done: by developing a behavioral focus on goals; including the patient's perspective even more (e.g., get Maria to talk about the details of relationships); developing an emotion focus (or a focus on the here and now); offering tentative interpretations (rather than finished formulations or too-open questions); unpacking micro-markers, such as specific words ("destroyed") and non- and paraverbal expressions (e.g., sighs, markers of contempt); offering help to the patient (but not assuming the patient necessarily wants the therapist's help); and by the therapist assuming their own limits in an interpersonally challenging situation. Most, if not all, strategies discussed here are focused on the here and now (as opposed to putting a relationship challenge explicitly within the developmental history of the patient). This may be a central feature for a therapist to effectively address the relationship challenges facing patients with personality disorders.

Addressing relationship challenges involves providing understanding and context that enable the patient to use the relationship in new and productive ways. We argue that this may serve two aims. First, addressing relationship challenges may serve as a relationship-building or management strategy, which seems needed in the case of Maria. Only with a solid groundwork of collaboration and mutual trust can this therapy start to address the core issues of this patient. Second, addressing relationship challenges in the manner described can act as a transformative force in itself. By working through relationship challenges within the therapeutic context, Maria can develop new patterns of relating and interacting that can contribute to her overall healing and growth. Again, given the case formulation, we assume this is central to Maria's case.

While each of our therapy models and intervention contexts may focus on one or several of the intervention best practices we discussed, we understand these are intervention strategies that foster an affective bond between the patient and therapist in the here and now as groundwork for further psychotherapy as a mutative relationship agent. Developing an affective bond, which involves overcoming relationship ruptures and deepening the emotional experience toward a more collaborative, transparent, immediate, true, trust-embedded, and authentic exchange, may be understood as a core mechanism of change. While there is necessarily a collaborative component in this mechanism, the affective bond may also be understood and studied from the patient's perspective alone. What patient processes indicate an affective bond and connection? When is the affective bond sufficiently strong or "good enough"? What does it mean for the patient to have a weak affective bond (vs. a strong affective bond vs. a sufficiently good one) with their therapist? What is the moment-by-moment fluctuation of the patient's affective bond with the therapist, and how important is it for the therapy overall? These questions, and more, may be addressed by future psychotherapy research.

10

DISCUSSING MECHANISMS OF CHANGE IN PSYCHOTHERAPIES FOR PERSONALITY DISORDERS

In this final chapter, we bring together the different threads discussed throughout the book. We synthesize what was learned by focusing on different levels of analysis, a variety of clinical and theoretical perspectives, and research on mechanisms of change in psychotherapies for personality disorders.

Although we know today that different psychotherapies work to effectively reduce symptoms and other problems related to personality disorders (see Budge et al., 2013; Storebø et al., 2020 for reviews), this research evidence is insufficient to adequately guide the clinician in daily practice. Treatment guidelines synthesize knowledge from the first level of analysis—a general treatment approach (as discussed in Chapter 1). Practice guidelines inform practicing clinicians about effective forms of treatment for specific pathological presentations. To translate research evidence into practice, results from randomized controlled trials and meta-analyses on borderline personality disorder (BPD) are readily available to guide decisions related to Level 1— a general approach that requires refinement. Level 2 focuses on predictors and

https://doi.org/10.1037/0000388-011
Understanding Mechanisms of Change in Psychotherapies for Personality Disorders, by U. Kramer, K. N. Levy, and S. McMain

moderators of treatment response and addresses the clinically important question of what works for whom.

What evidence is there to support the hypothesis that individual patient profiles are associated with different treatment responses? We found that certain profiles of patients with BPD—such as comorbidity with complex trauma, adolescence, high symptom severity, and agreeableness—are associated with better therapy outcomes (e.g., Keefe et al., 2020). Taken together, the research from the first two levels is an initial step toward personalizing psychotherapy for patients with personality disorders, but much more work needs to be done. More research is needed to understand how to tailor psychotherapy approaches and strategies to particular patients and specific moments in therapy.

Level 3 (from Chapter 1) describes the mechanisms of change in psychotherapy, which is the core contribution of this book. It is central to understanding why psychotherapy works and how, which may be articulated with the clinically relevant Level 4 related to case formulation. A key aspect of focusing on mechanisms of change in psychotherapy is that we are interested in what changes in the person that moves them toward mental health (as opposed to a focus on psychopathology and its mechanisms). This involves some level of hopefulness that, under certain conditions and processes, personality pathology will diminish over time and appropriate treatment, and life can be reclaimed (Gunderson & Hoffman, 2016). Salutogenic processes are at play in any helpful human interaction; mechanisms of change are such processes that specifically act in the context of psychological treatments, bringing about positive change in the patients' lives.

While we are enthusiastic about the growing interest in developing a research base to determine what processes account for change in psychotherapy outcomes, the findings to date provide only a limited understanding of such mechanisms of change. Given this duality between the huge potential and the limits in our present knowledge, we structure our discussion as a byproduct of theory, research, and clinical expertise. We begin with a general summary statement and a set of hypotheses to be tested by strong and internationally coordinated research programs and experienced clinicians seeking to focus on fostering mechanisms of change in the treatment of patients with personality disorders. Next, we continue with a section on methodological advances in the study of these mechanisms of change. This latter section is a road map for psychotherapy researchers interested in going further, exploring, and testing some of the hypotheses identified in this book.

PATHS TO CHANGE IN PSYCHOTHERAPIES FOR PERSONALITY DISORDERS

In this section, we synthesize the six paths to change discussed in Chapters 4 through 9. We begin by considering relationship challenges because they provide a general context for understanding the process of change in the five functional domains, as shown in Figure 10.1.

As with all models of psychotherapy, the development of an individualized case formulation is a critical step to understanding an individual case. A sound case formulation is especially important when attempting to make sense of highly complex individuals with personality disorders who are prone to behave

FIGURE 10.1. Overview of Paths to Change in Psychotherapies for Personality Disorders

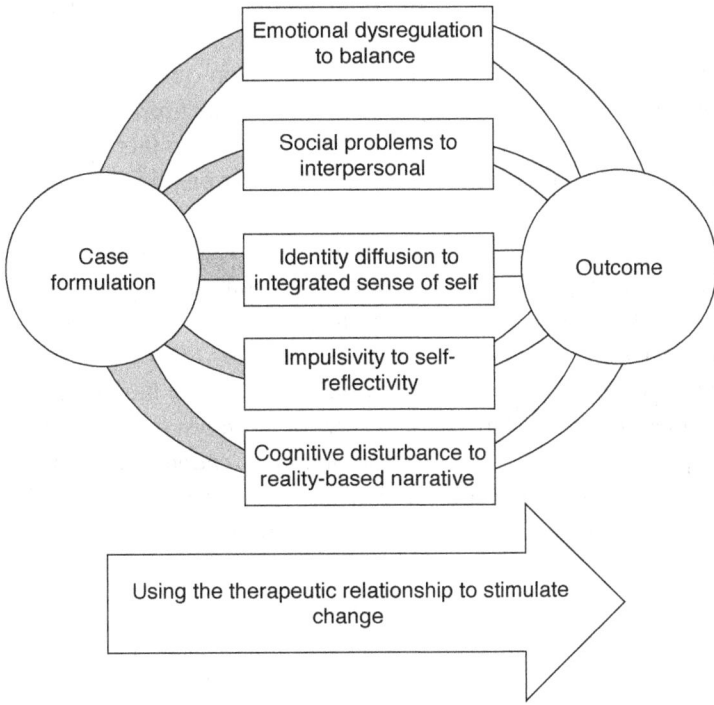

Note. Case formulation is relevant during the therapy process and determines both the selection of a focus on a functional domain and the type of relationship experience that would help stimulate change in a particular case. Focusing on the therapeutic relationship is also important throughout the whole process. Note that the process does not follow a fully linear path as implied by this image, and overlap between the five other paths of change is expected.

differently in different states. Case formulation involves distilling theory and providing a comprehensive account of the range of problems and relevant elements of a particular case through the formulation model. A case formulation helps to explain how seemingly disparate problematic behaviors and experiences are related by drawing inferences between behaviors. A sound case formulation helps therapists determine the most productive therapeutic focus (one of the first five paths to change; the sixth path focusing on relationship challenges is always involved), the optimal relational stance, and what types of interventions would be most effective for a specific individual. It will also help navigate the therapeutic relationship and specific choice points in the treatment.

Using the Therapeutic Relationship to Foster Change

The impact of the therapeutic relationship on patient outcomes is widely acknowledged across various therapeutic approaches. However, establishing and maintaining a positive therapeutic relationship can be particularly challenging in psychotherapy for individuals with personality disorders. While all therapy models recognize the importance of a positive therapeutic relationship, they differ in their views on whether the strength of the relationship alone is sufficient for producing therapeutic change.

In transference-focused psychotherapy (TFP), for instance, therapists conceptualize and emphasize challenges in the therapeutic relationship by linking them to the patient's object relations playing out in the current therapy dynamic. However, in dialectical behavior therapy (DBT), a positive therapeutic relationship is considered essential. The dialectic lies in the belief that the therapeutic relationship itself can serve as a catalyst for change by activating the patient's inherent wisdom and adaptive tendencies. Simultaneously, the therapist's role within this relationship becomes a means of influencing the therapy process. In line with a comprehensive case formulation, therapists working within a motive-oriented therapeutic relationship approach explicitly aim to cultivate a corrective relationship experience. This is done through various tailored strategies specific to each individual and adaptable to different stages of the therapeutic process, all in alignment with the case formulation.

From this perspective, the therapist's responses are guided by an individualized understanding of the patient and adjusted according to the specific needs and circumstances that arise throughout the therapy journey. By flexibly choosing how to respond in each moment, the therapist maximizes the potential for creating a therapeutic relationship that fosters positive change in the patient.

In working with a patient like Maria (Chapter 9), who presents with multiple challenges in the therapeutic relationship (i.e., nonverbal expression of contempt and other negative affect, criticisms of the previous therapy, extremely fragile self-presentation, and expressed doubt about therapy's helpfulness and hostility), it may be useful for a therapist to take into account each of these diverse conceptualizations and related intervention strategies. There was a consensus that therapy would be successful if the therapist nurtures the patient's sense of safety and trust in the therapist. This can be achieved if the therapist responds with higher levels of validation, especially in response to the patient's affective experience, by providing sensitive clarifying statements rather than extensive questioning and by helping stimulate the patient's innate potential, vision, and goals. A particularly effective means of intervention to promote relationship safety includes a focus on Maria's emotional experience (Greenberg, 2019) and helping her unpack and differentiate highly charged words (e.g., "I am destroyed") within the current context.

Another point of consensus is the significance of focusing on the present moment within the therapeutic relationship. The challenges experienced in the relationship serve as triggers for underlying core issues that exist within both the client and, to some extent, the therapist (Eubanks et al., 2022; Muran & Eubanks, 2020). These relationship challenges, as observed in the case of this patient, likely stem from interpersonal patterns or schemas that have developed through the patient's social environment and personal history (Smith et al., 2020). Activating such interpersonal behaviors during therapy sessions may be necessary to modify deeply ingrained relationship memory structures. In certain therapeutic approaches, these activated behaviors are referred to as *testing behaviors* (Silberschatz, 2005).

By activating the underlying problematic schematic memory, with specific contents related to the self and self in relation to others (e.g., beliefs of rejection or lack of value), the stage is set for facilitating change (Grawe, 1998; Lane et al., 2015; Smith et al., 2020). Insights from memory reconsolidation research have suggested that activating an old memory places it in a temporarily malleable state, making it open to change when new and inconsistent information becomes available (Smith et al., 2020). From this perspective, a patient grappling with relationship difficulties is taking a significant step toward productive change. Maria's activation of self, other, and relational schemas represents the first crucial phase. If the therapist responds appropriately, the patient's awareness of these relationship patterns in the present moment can be heightened, allowing for a revision and update of assumptions based on current reality (Smith et al., 2020).

The subsequent step involves generalizing the learning that has taken place within the therapy relationship to other relationships outside the therapy room. This process entails applying the insights gained and skills developed within therapy to real-life interactions with others. By doing so, Maria can foster positive changes in her relational dynamics beyond the confines of the therapeutic setting.

From Emotion Dysregulation to Emotion Balance

The change pathway with the strongest empirical evidence across various psychotherapy approaches is enhancing emotion regulation. Nevertheless, many questions remain unaddressed (see Chapter 4). Consistent with the literature, Marcus (the patient from Chapter 4's case example) presented with various choice points related to deficits in emotion dysregulation triggered by interpersonal situations. Even when the patient was alone, his unmodulated anger and impulsive texting were triggered by his relationship problems with Laura, his girlfriend who had recently broken up with him. Interpersonal relatedness is fundamental to emotional needs. This underscores the importance of clinicians assessing (a) the precise interpersonal trigger to the episode of emotion dysregulation and (b) the core emotion response (i.e., bodily felt sensations, body physiology, emotions, cognitions, action urges). We agreed that tools such as DBT's behavioral chain analysis could be helpful not only in the context of DBT but also as a tool to be integrated into other psychotherapy approaches because it deepens the understanding of the core emotion processes in relation to interpersonal relationships (Sonley & Choi-Kain, 2021). Depending on the task, a large variety of techniques from diverse therapy approaches can be useful at this juncture of the psychotherapy.

For example, the therapist may foster the patient's insight into the links between self-criticism and feelings of shame, emptiness, and loneliness. The therapist may also focus on the patient's emotions to help them differentiate their emotional experience. This can include fostering awareness of body sensations, differentiating secondary and primary emotions, and "hot teaching" content and skills. The interpersonal context of emotion dysregulation requires (as in Marcus's first choice point) the patient's uptake of specific GIVE skills (be gentle, act interested, validate, and use an easy manner) or the increased use of social relationships as resources, which may be explicitly fostered by the therapist.

It is interesting to note that many, if not all, psychotherapy models working with patients with BPD offer something to help move from emotion dysregulation to emotion balance. It is up to each psychotherapist to use the tools that are (a) most consistent with the specific individual's case formulation and (b) at the therapist's disposal (due to specific resources, training, or preference;

see Table 4.1). We highlight that some emotion regulation strategies develop in the therapy implicitly and explicitly. For example, while modeling can be explicit, it also occurs implicitly (e.g., latent learning) or through physiological synchrony.

From Problems in Social Interaction to Interpersonal Effectiveness

Addressing dysfunction in social interactions is a prominent characteristic of personality disorders, making the enhancement of relationships a crucial objective in psychotherapy. Extensive research has provided solid evidence supporting the effectiveness of interventions aimed at improving interpersonal functioning (Bateman & Fonagy, 2009; Clarkin, Levy, et al., 2007; McMain et al., 2009), although further investigation is still warranted. Chapter 5 delved into the case of Janet, which demonstrated the use of multiple avenues to foster change in her pursuit of interpersonal effectiveness.

Difficulties in social interaction may not only be present in real life but also the therapeutic interaction, thus becoming a relationship challenge (see the previous section on the therapeutic relationship and Chapter 9). The latter observation may put therapists in difficult situations at times. For example, when the therapist has to choose the depth of a comment, they may have to understand in detail what is happening in the interaction. Here, different approaches may be helpful to different folks (Blatt & Felsen, 1993). The depth of a therapist intervention (i.e., the therapist directly addressing the links between the past interpersonal relationship serving as a blueprint for the current problematic interaction with the therapist vs. the therapist addressing any other issues before such interventions) may be a function of the perceived quality of the therapeutic relationship and the quality of the patient's current emotional state. A patient working within a globally positive therapeutic relationship and capable of modulating intense anger or frustration may be more receptive and ready to assimilate the therapist's interventions than a patient who struggles to trust the therapist. If interpersonal trust is an issue for the patient, therapist cautiousness may be recommended, but we recommend these assumptions be tested by further research.

From Identity Diffusion to an Integrated Sense of Self

Moving from an unintegrated sense of self to a more consolidated and affirmed identity may also account for positive outcomes in psychotherapy for personality disorders. Patients with personality pathology often present with unclear boundaries between self and others, with a lack of direction and an opposing, unintegrated view of themself. As seen in Chapter 6 in the case of Leon, the therapist used a variety of interventions, such as expressing confusion and challenging perceptions in the context of conflicting patient presentations, using metaphors, focusing on the patient's emotional experience, and validating the truly valid. Depending on whether the case formulation stresses representational, affective, or motivational origins of the diffused identity, the therapist may intervene differently in each case. The therapist may interpret the underlying conflict between representations, increase awareness of the potential polarization within the self, or choose to ground their intervention in the overarching motives behind the conflicting aspects of the self. As in the case of Leon, the therapist may need to slow the process down to help the patient become aware of the implications of their behavior and generate new meaning. The therapist may help the patient become more aware of the underlying affect and what they are seeking from therapy. These interventions may give the patient direction without offering direct solutions to the patient's dilemma. We agree among us that an identity-diffused patient needs a tactful and responsive psychotherapist who, at times, is a half step behind and, at other times, a half step in front of the patient in the microprocess of therapy. We also agree that the therapist should constantly be willing to question the appropriateness of what they are doing. Balancing opposing constraints— avoiding both therapist passivity and content directiveness—may be key to fostering a more affirmative and integrated sense of self in the patient.

From Impulsive Behaviors to Self-Reflectivity

The transition from impulsive behaviors to a reflective stance regarding oneself and relationships is a pivotal mechanism of change in the treatment of personality disorders. This transformative process requires a combination of insight-focused interventions to enhance awareness of the impact of impulsive behaviors on the self and relationships, as well as skills-focused interventions to foster mindfulness, emotional awareness, and distress tolerance.

When impulsive expressions arise during therapy sessions, it is vital to approach them from two complementary perspectives. First, addressing impulsivity requires therapists to prioritize trust and cooperation to eliminate destructive behaviors. Second, it is crucial to establish a structure within therapy sessions to address impulsivity effectively. This may entail gently redirecting the patient's focus and ensuring they remain aligned with their short- and long-term goals. Therapist validation and support are crucial in guiding this process. However, discerning the validity of a patient's experiences can be complex because distinguishing between what is reasonable and what is not may prove challenging. In such cases, the therapist can rely on case formulation, seek peer support, and engage in clinical supervision to navigate situations where patient impulsivity is prevalent.

Chapter 7 provided an illustrative example of the therapist's interventions and the patient's journey from impulsivity to reflectiveness. It highlighted how the therapist's strategic actions facilitate this transformative process and emphasized the significance of the patient's pathway in developing a more thoughtful and considered approach to their thoughts, emotions, and interpersonal dynamics.

The focus on the functional domain of impulsivity is a high-priority task in the treatment of individuals with personality disorders. The domain of impulsivity is closely linked to the alternative model of personality disorders dimensional construct of disinhibition (American Psychiatric Association, 2022), which subsumes patient acting out, suicidal and homicidal threats and actions, and aggressiveness. For the latter (i.e., aggressive behavior), a specific integrative modular treatment has been developed and assessed from a mechanisms-based perspective (Herpertz et al., 2021). As such, reducing aggressive behavior represents one of the more empirically validated paths to change in the treatment of personality disorders. Nonetheless, more research will be needed to illuminate the step-by-step move from impulsive behaviors to a more self-reflective stance. This research may focus on (a) the patient shifting in-session emotional arousal; (b) the therapist offering relational attributes, including nonjudgment, validation, and genuineness (i.e., self-disclosure) to build and strengthen the patient's engagement; (c) the patient's increasing awareness of the behavior underlying nonproblematic motives; (d) the patient's increasing awareness of the triggers of behavioral impulsivity; and (e) the patient's increasing awareness of the interpersonal consequences of dysregulated states.

From Cognitive Disturbance to a Coherent and Reality-Based Narrative

The path to change associated with the final functional domain overlaps with specific diagnostic criteria (i.e., Criteria 9 of BPD according to the *Diagnostic and Statistical Manual of Mental Disorders*, 5th ed., text rev. [*DSM-5-TR*]; American Psychiatric Association, 2022). While this may prove to be complicated from a research perspective (i.e., with the difficulty of disentangling the process from the outcome, as discussed later), it may not pose more difficulties clinically. From the latter perspective, it appears from Chapter 8 that a careful diagnosis will help circumscribe the phenomenon in detail, then treat it accurately, tactfully, and directly. A direct and prominent focus on the reality distortion (or the delusional belief, as in Irene's case from Chapter 8) by offering a mix of genuine interest, grounding in the here and now, and support in the development of wise-mind and clarifying triggers may help support the patient in gently moving toward a more coherent and reality-based narrative. On the road to achieving this, the patient may have to examine the veracity of the belief, be able to decrease their emotional arousal in the moment, but also allow emotion to come up and become aware of triggers. Related to this direct and prominent focus on the reality distortion, there may be other issues that the therapist needs to address (such as in the case of Irene): fostering the integration of opposing views or helping the patient make hard decisions for their life.

The Timing and the Complexity of Interventions Facing Patients With Personality Pathology

Severe forms of personality pathology may be diagnosed more precisely in the future using the dimensional construct of Criterion A of the alternative model of personality disorders of the *DSM-5-TR* or the severity index in the *International Statistical Classification of Diseases and Related Health Problems* (11th ed.; World Health Organization, 2022). Both conceptions do not specify which symptoms the severe forms are associated with, but research has suggested that specific acute symptoms from the borderline spectrum, if present, may be optimal predictors of severe forms of personality pathology: frequent impulsivity, frequent and severe self-harm, and frequent suicidal or homicidal thoughts and actions (e.g., Bach et al., 2022; Clark et al., 2017). These symptoms may also be considered the most difficult for therapists to deal with and are prominent in predicting treatment failures from the first session on (see our clinical recommendations in Chapter 3). When discussing these manifestations associated with particularly severe forms of personality disorders, it becomes clear that timing is key. Also, what may work for one patient may not necessarily be helpful for another. For these reasons, when faced with these manifestations (see Chapters 6, 7, and 8 for clinical examples), the therapist needs to make an assessment to help them to decide whether (a) this patient poses a threat to life or integrity (to themselves or others) or (b) this patient does not pose a threat to life or integrity but may pose such a threat sometime in the future. According to this assessment, the therapist offers (a) crisis management, which may involve what a TFP therapist would call technical neutrality, and straightforward help to overcome the current threat or crisis in a matter-of-fact manner and (b) interventions that are consistent with the previously described six mechanisms of change, depending on the case formulation, preventing the threat from materializing in the future.

We demonstrated that each functional domain as starting point for a mechanism of change in treatments for personality disorder is not independent; we expect overlap between the functional domains because they are not orthogonal dimensions in understanding personality pathology. Figure 10.1. may falsely suggest that the different paths to change are like railroads on which change is produced linearly, and no deviation or unexpected opportunity for change may arise in the form of a clinical choice point. This is not the case in psychotherapy, which corresponds more to navigating a maze. Such navigation may involve the therapist selecting several sequential paths or parts of paths to change to help the patient get better. We do not exclude that the model presented here may be simplified in the future and entail fewer and more general mechanisms of change. Conversely, as research gets more detailed in this domain we can also imagine that this model may become more complex and detailed, involving many more effective paths.

METHODOLOGICAL CONSIDERATIONS AND FUTURE DIRECTIONS FOR PSYCHOTHERAPY RESEARCH ON MECHANISMS OF CHANGE IN PERSONALITY PATHOLOGY

Throughout this book, we have observed that no mechanism of change has explained outcomes in psychotherapy for personality disorders when applying the strict criteria outlined by Kazdin (2009; see Chapter 1). While there is slightly more evidence for the efficacy of treatments for other psychological problems, such as exposure therapies for anxiety disorders, where in-session fear activation and between-session habituation has been shown to function as mechanisms of change (Crits-Christoph & Connolly Gibbons, 2021), the majority of studies on treatments for personality pathology remain correlational (Crits-Christoph & Connolly Gibbons, 2021; Kramer, Beuchat, et al., 2020). These correlational studies observe associations between in-session patient processes and symptom change, but the directionality of the relationship and the influence of third variables are unclear.

It is also impossible to rule out the influence of third variables explaining the effects. Other limitations involve the limited value of a process that is highly specific to a particular therapy approach, the lack of modeling of the effects related to therapist responsiveness, the lack of modeling of the nesting of patients within therapists, the lack of modeling the interaction between the effect of a therapist intervention and the patient's uptake of this intervention (see also therapist responsiveness; Crits-Christoph & Connolly Gibbons, 2021; Stiles et al., 1998), the lack of measurement of out-of-session mechanisms (see the differentiation by Doss, 2004), and the lack of measurement of central biological correlates of change mechanisms.

Another problem in the classical process-outcome design is often the dependability of a measure. Assessing the therapeutic alliance at different sessions or therapy phases introduces variability, and the meaning of assessment items may depend on the timing of the assessment. As a reflection of the beginning status of our field of mechanisms of change in psychotherapy, another problem involves the general constructs used by researchers (i.e., "therapeutic alliance," "emotion regulation," or "mentalization") that are of little true value in understanding event-based sequential components of what works in therapy (and what does not). We think that a more fine-grained and event-based conceptualization, such as those proposed in this book, can readily translate into clinical recommendations for what the therapist should do when facing a patient-related choice point.

Clearly, a push for methodological improvement in the study of mechanisms of change and a focus on personality disorders is needed because the demonstration of change in facets associated with personality (and personality disorders) may be among the core tasks of psychotherapy research (Kramer, Eubanks, et al., 2022). Personality pathology conceptualized within five multilevel functional domains may underlie, to various degrees, many symptom presentations of patients in psychotherapy. As such, activated behaviors associated with one (or more) of these five functional domains represent opportunities for change and become priority intervention targets. Thus, the six resulting pathways outlined previously may serve as starting points for research.

With the experimental demonstration of a phenomenon being the ultimate proof of evidence, psychotherapy researchers have successfully translated statistical methods from agronomics (Fisher, 1935) into randomization for psychotherapy outcome research, which should provide relatively convincing arguments for the causality of the effect of an intervention. However, as we saw in Chapter 1, this strategy is not always sufficient for outcome research and even less so for patient-related mechanisms of change that cannot be randomly attributed to a condition by a computer program.

Demonstrating causality is steeped in theory and specific tenets or predictions related to a theory (Morgan & Winship, 2008; Pearls et al., 2016; Pearls & Mackenzie, 2020). Hypotheses formulated earlier about paths to change in personality pathology (see Figure 10.1) may be useful. The researcher should be willing to make a graphical model of the presumed links between the concepts and the orientation of these links to model a causal effect. A more detailed, step-by-step process should be devised for each path to change discussed here. A full causal model may be outlined previously where we assume that six paths to change in personality pathology potentially cause a change in symptoms (as defined as outcome in a psychotherapy trial).

Intensive assessments of all components of the model across time in psychotherapy are needed to test the model outlined in this book or parts of it. Here, intensive means both multimethod and more than twice over time. In addition, as Pearls and Mackenzie (2020) discussed, only including all potentially (causally) influential variables will yield a sufficiently complete model that can rule out confounding factors. Psychotherapy researchers often continue to only assess, if at all, a preferred mechanism of change and fail to develop and test a fuller model involving all potentially causal variables.

For example, to test the within-person effect of moving from emotion dysregulation to emotion balance according to a decrease in borderline symptoms at the end of psychotherapy, researchers need to assess at multiple time points (e.g., after each therapy session or from one minute to the next within the session) both event-based aspects of emotional regulation (or emotion processing) and borderline symptoms. In this fashion, a causal model can be devised to explain the effect of change in emotional processing at Session number n-lagged − 1 (i.e., one session before Session n) on reducing borderline symptoms at Session n. In this model, consistent with the six-pathway model, it is necessary to test alternative paths to change to reach firm conclusions related to the specificity of an effect associated with event-based emotion processing. Session-by-session changes may overlook the theoretically and clinically relevant opportunities for change. A more detailed examination of the process involves studying sequential changes in emotion from one minute to the next, using a similar within-person effect approach but within a shorter time. The challenge here may be to develop assessments of the outcomes at a similar time scale, although physiological measures of outcomes may be a productive way to move forward.

To address the dependability of the measurement and the lack of specificity in some constructs—the within-person fluctuation of an evolving process over time—the researcher can, according to their theory, select an event (Rice & Greenberg, 1984) that is most likely to produce the manifestation of the mechanism of interest. In this book, such an event is consistent with the notion of the clinical choice point. For example, in the case of Marcus from Chapter 4, who presented with high levels of self-criticism, the researcher may select from videos and analyze only moments of the therapy when such self-criticism is expressed. The event-related and clinically relevant mechanism of change would become the emotion in response to self-criticism. If the emotional response to this event is assessed multiple times over the course of therapy and change can be demonstrated, the changing emotion in response to self-criticism can be tested in regard to the effects of the psychotherapy. In addition to addressing the dependability problem of the measurement, research that focuses on significant events would also narrow the gap between research and clinical practice because event-based psychotherapy research will arguably yield conclusions such as "if–then," which are most helpful for informing clinicians what to do when.

Another perspective offers a differentiation between the notion of process and mechanism of change. Doss (2004) differentiated between (a) therapist interventions (see Tables 4.1–8.1, which present generic and approach-specific interventions separately), (b) in-session patient processes (i.e., as a response to the therapist intervention; see the patient processes in Tables 4.1–8.1), and (c) the patient's change mechanisms (i.e., defined in this framework as out-of-session skills or processes explaining symptom decrease). To take into account these distinctions, intensive evaluations of the in-session processes and real-life mechanisms and symptoms are required. For example, a researcher interested in studying the paths to change from problematic social interaction to interpersonal effectiveness could implement daily assessments on the patient's phone using ecological momentary assessment to observe social behaviors adopted in interpersonally stressful situations (i.e., interactions with a significant other) and in-situ patient awareness of the interaction, in addition to in-session observation of the patient's mentalizing capacities and outcomes. Again, the researcher would use a within-person analysis to explain the outcomes by the lagged −1 (or −*n*) change in the different operationalizations (within and between sessions) of interpersonal effectiveness. In a causal model, the between-session observations should be predicted by interactions in the therapy hour (i.e., specific therapist interventions and responding patient processes) preceding this day-to-day assessment of interpersonal effectiveness and personality outcomes.

It is valuable to include physiological or neurofunctional assessments to incorporate the biological underpinnings of change in personality pathology (Kramer, Eubanks, et al., 2022). For instance, in studying the transition from impulsive behaviors to self-reflection, a researcher could assess the patient's saliva cortisol levels multiple times during therapy sessions as biomarkers of sympathetic nervous system activity associated with physiological arousal. By using a within-person design with repeated assessments of both biological and psychological measures related to the problem behavior (e.g., antisocial symptoms or the impulsivity subscale of the Zanarini Rating Scale for BPD; Zanarini et al., 1989), these factors can be sequentially integrated into a model predicting the outcome of psychotherapy. This approach allows for a comprehensive examination of the relationship between biological markers, psychological processes, and treatment outcomes.

In addition to controlling for therapist responsiveness in statistical analysis, another approach is to adopt an "if–then" model that embraces momentary conditional interventions (Kramer, Eubanks, et al., 2022). In this approach, the researcher can identify specific choice points associated with each path to change discussed in this book and instruct therapists to implement targeted interventions based on those moments. These interventions would be implemented if the choice point reflected an activated patient behavior related to a functional domain or specific challenge in the therapy relationship and if the case formulation and clinical theory supported the intervention at that moment. Comparing this "if–then responsive-to-the-patient" approach with a standard therapy approach for personality pathology could provide experimental evidence of the impact of therapist responsiveness on the course and outcomes of treatment for patients with personality disorders. This type of demonstration holds the potential to strengthen our understanding of the role of therapist responsiveness in therapeutic effectiveness.

A few studies have incorporated the aforementioned designs to investigate mechanisms of change in psychotherapy for personality disorders. For example, in the study by Herpertz et al. (2021), the effect of an integrative treatment module focusing on aggressive behavior as part of the impulsivity functional domain was assessed using a randomized controlled design. In this study, the treatment explicitly focused on mechanisms and improving an area of function in patients with BPD. As suggested earlier, the study also applied a multimethod approach to assessing the mediators by incorporating behavioral and neurofunctional assessments over time. Another example is the study by Babl et al. (2022), which examined a large naturalistic sample of psychotherapy for personality disorders. A mediation model tested the sequential influence of patient in-session problematic interpersonal patterns and therapist interventions in response to these patterns, showing a step-by-time time-dependent mediation of insight-increasing therapeutic interventions explaining outcomes. A final example is the study by Kivity et al. (2021), in which therapist interventions focusing on reflective functioning in TFP were assessed in session and analyzed with regard to in-session emotion arousal in an event-based step-by-step manner explaining outcomes.

Our hope is that our consolidated synthesis of mechanisms of change in psychotherapies for personality disorders will enhance the precision of psychotherapy to help even more patients to a greater degree and depth, enabling them to achieve lifelong lasting change. We observe that our attempt to understand mechanisms of change in psychotherapy for personality disorders had a beginning and an end (at least for now), had depth and shallowness, moments of frustration (about possible stalemates in the dialogue) and pleasure (about the discovery of a new idea in the dialogue), and most of all, has brought us closer together as human beings. We hope the result will stimulate the field to move toward clinical excellence and more research focusing on understanding mechanisms of change for patients with personality disorders.

References

Allport, G. W. (1937). *Personality: A psychological interpretation*. Holt.

American Psychiatric Association. (1968). *Diagnostic and statistical manual of mental disorders* (2nd ed.). https://dsm.psychiatryonline.org/doi/epdf/10.1176/appi. books.9780890420355.dsm-ii

American Psychiatric Association. (1980). *Diagnostic and statistical manual of mental disorders* (3rd ed.).

American Psychiatric Association. (2022). *Diagnostic and statistical manual of mental disorders* (5th ed., text rev.). https://doi.org/10.1176/appi.books. 9780890425787

Anderson, T., Knobloch-Fedders, L. M., Stiles, W. B., Ordoñez, T., & Heckman, B. D. (2012). The power of subtle interpersonal hostility in psychodynamic psychotherapy: A speech acts analysis. *Psychotherapy Research*, *22*(3), 348–362. https://doi.org/10.1080/10503307.2012.658097

Angus, L. E., Boritz, T., Bryntwick, E., Carpenter, N., Macaulay, C., & Khattra, J. (2017). The Narrative-Emotion Process Coding System 2.0: A multi-methodological approach to identifying and assessing narrative-emotion process markers in psychotherapy. *Psychotherapy Research*, *27*(3), 253–269. https://doi.org/10.1080/ 10503307.2016.1238525

Angus, L. E., Boritz, T., Mendes, I., & Gonçalves, M. M. (2019). Narrative change processes and patient treatment outcomes in emotion-focused therapy. In L. S. Greenberg & R. N. Goldman (Eds.), *Clinical handbook of emotion-focused therapy* (pp. 243–260). American Psychological Association. https://doi.org/ 10.1037/0000112-011

Arntz, A., Hawke, L. D., Bamelis, L., Spinhoven, P., & Molendijk, M. L. (2012). Changes in natural language use as an indicator of psychotherapeutic change in personality disorders. *Behaviour Research and Therapy*, *50*(3), 191–202. https://doi.org/10.1016/j.brat.2011.12.007

Babl, A., Berger, T., Eubanks, C. F., Gómez Penedo, J. M., Caspar, F., Sachse, R., & Kramer, U. (2022). Addressing interpersonal patterns in patients with personality disorders partially explains psychotherapy outcome via changes in interaction patterns: A mediation analysis. *Psychotherapy Research, 32*(8), 984–994. Advance online publication. https://doi.org/10.1080/10503307.2022.2036383

Bach, B., Kerber, A., Aluja, A., Bastiaens, T., Keeley, J. W., Claes, L., Fossati, A., Gutierrez, F., Oliveira, S. E. S., Pires, R., Riegel, K. D., Rolland, J. P., Roskam, I., Sellbom, M., Somma, A., Spanemberg, L., Strus, W., Thimm, J. C., Wright, A. G. C., & Zimmermann, J. (2020). International assessment of *DSM-5* and *ICD-11* personality disorder traits: Toward a common nosology in DSM-5.1. *Psychopathology, 53*(3–4), 179–188. https://doi.org/10.1159/000507589

Bach, B., Kramer, U., Doering, S., di Giacomo, E., Hutsebaut, J., Kaera, A., De Panfilis, C., Schmahl, C., Swales, M., Taubner, S., & Renneberg, B. (2022). The *ICD-11* classification of personality disorders: A European perspective on challenges and opportunities. *Borderline Personality Disorder and Emotion Dysregulation, 9*, Article 12. https://doi.org/10.1186/s40479-022-00182-0

Baer, R. A., Smith, G. T., & Allen, K. B. (2004). Assessment of mindfulness by self-report: The Kentucky Inventory of Mindfulness Skills. *Assessment, 11*(3), 191–206. https://doi.org/10.1177/1073191104268029

Bari, A. B., Kellermann, T. S., & Studer, B. (2016). Impulsiveness and inhibitory mechanisms. In J. R. Absher & J. Cloutier (Eds.), *Neuroimaging personality, social cognition and character* (pp. 113–136). Academic Press. https://doi.org/10.1016/B978-0-12-800935-2.00006-3

Barkham, M., & Lambert, M. J. (2021). The efficacy and effectiveness of psychological therapies. In M. Barkham, W. Lutz, & L. G. Castonguay (Eds.), *Bergin and Garfield's handbook of psychotherapy and behavior change: 50th anniversary edition* (pp. 135–189). Wiley.

Barnicot, K., Katsakou, C., Bhatti, N., Savill, M., Fearns, N., & Priebe, S. (2012). Factors predicting the outcome of psychotherapy for borderline personality disorder: A systematic review. *Clinical Psychology Review, 32*(5), 400–412. https://doi.org/10.1016/j.cpr.2012.04.004

Bartz, J. A., Zaki, J., Bolger, N., & Ochsner, K. N. (2011). Social effects of oxytocin in humans: Context and person matter. *Trends in Cognitive Sciences, 15*(7), 301–309. Advance online publication. https://doi.org/10.1016/j.tics.2011.05.002

Bateman, A., & Fonagy, P. (2006). Mentalizing and borderline personality disorder. In J. G. Allen & P. Fonagy (Eds.), *Handbook of mentalization-based treatment* (pp. 183–200). Wiley. https://doi.org/10.1002/9780470712986.ch9

Bateman, A., & Fonagy, P. (2009). Randomized controlled trial of outpatient mentalization-based treatment versus structured clinical management for borderline personality disorder. *The American Journal of Psychiatry, 166*(12), 1355–1364. https://doi.org/10.1176/appi.ajp.2009.09040539

Bateman, A., & Fonagy, P. (2015). *Mentalization-based treatment for borderline personality disorder: A practical guide.* Oxford University Press. https://doi.org/10.1093/med/9780198570905.001.0001

Beblo, T., Fernando, S., Kamper, P., Griepenstroh, J., Aschenbrenner, S., Pastuszak, A., Schlosser, N., & Driessen, M. (2013). Increased attempts to suppress negative and positive emotions in borderline personality disorder. *Psychiatry Research*, *210*(2), 505–509. https://doi.org/10.1016/j.psychres.2013.06.036

Bedics, J. D., Atkins, D. C., Comtois, K. A., & Linehan, M. M. (2012). Treatment differences in the therapeutic relationship and introject during a 2-year randomized controlled trial of dialectical behavior therapy versus nonbehavioral psychotherapy experts for borderline personality disorder. *Journal of Consulting and Clinical Psychology*, *80*(1), 66–77. https://doi.org/10.1037/a0026113

Beeney, J. E., Stepp, S. D., Hallquist, M. N., Scott, L. N., Wright, A. G. C., Ellison, W. D., Nolf, K. A., & Pilkonis, P. A. (2015). Attachment and social cognition in borderline personality disorder: Specificity in relation to antisocial and avoidant personality disorders. *Personality Disorders*, *6*(3), 207–215. https://doi.org/10.1037/per0000110

Berenson, K. R., Downey, G., Rafaeli, E., Coifman, K. G., & Paquin, N. L. (2011). The rejection-rage contingency in borderline personality disorder. *Journal of Abnormal Psychology*, *120*(3), 681–690. https://doi.org/10.1037/a0023335

Berenson, K. R., Gyurak, A., Downey, G., Ayduk, O., Mogg, K., Bradley, B., & Pine, D. (2013). *Rejection Sensitivity Questionnaire, Adult version (A-RSQ)*. https://berenson.sites.gettysburg.edu/wp-content/uploads/2018/02/ARSQ-scoring-1.pdf

Berkman, L. F., & Syme, S. L. (1979). Social networks, host resistance, and mortality: A nine-year follow-up study of Alameda County residents. *American Journal of Epidemiology*, *109*(2), 186–204. https://doi.org/10.1093/oxfordjournals.aje.a112674

Bernstein, J., Zimmerman, M., & Auchincloss, E. L. (2015). Transference-focused psychotherapy training during residency: An aide to learning psychodynamic psychotherapy. *Psychodynamic Psychiatry*, *43*(2), 201–221. https://doi.org/10.1521/pdps.2015.43.2.201

Berthoud, L., Pascual-Leone, A., Caspar, F., Tissot, H., Keller, S., Rohde, K. B., de Roten, Y., Despland, J. N., & Kramer, U. (2017). Leaving distress behind: A randomized controlled study on change in emotional processing in borderline personality disorder. *Psychiatry*, *80*(2), 139–154. https://doi.org/10.1080/00332747.2016.1220230

Bertsch, K., Koenigsberg, H., Niedtfeld, I., & Schmahl, C. (2018). Emotion regulation. In C. Schmahl, K. Luan Phan, R. O. Friedel, & L. J. Siever (Eds.), *Neurobiology of personality disorders* (pp. 133–156). Oxford University Press.

Bland, A. R., & Rossen, E. K. (2005). Clinical supervision of nurses working with patients with borderline personality disorder. *Issues in Mental Health Nursing*, *26*(5), 507–517. https://doi.org/10.1080/01612840590931957

Blatt, S., & Felsen, I. (1993). "Different kinds of folks may need different kinds of strokes": The effect of patients' characteristics on therapeutic process and outcome. *Psychotherapy Research, 3*(4), 245–259. https://doi.org/10.1080/10503309312331333829

Bleuler, E. (1911). *Dementia praecox oder Gruppe der Schizophrenien* [Dementia praecox or the group of schizophrenias]. Deuticke.

Bohus, M., Schmahl, C., Fydrich, T., Steil, R., Müller-Engelmann, M., Herzog, J., Ludäscher, P., Kleindienst, N., & Priebe, K. (2019). A research programme to evaluate DBT-PTSD, a modular treatment approach for Complex PTSD after childhood abuse. *Borderline Personality Disorder and Emotion Dysregulation, 6*(1), 7. Advance online publication. https://doi.org/10.1186/s40479-019-0099-y

Boritz, T., Barnhart, R., Angus, L., & Constantino, M. J. (2017). Narrative flexibility in brief psychotherapy for depression. *Psychotherapy Research, 27*(6), 666–676. https://doi.org/10.1080/10503307.2016.1152410

Boritz, T., Barnhart, R., Eubanks, C. F., & McMain, S. (2018). Alliance rupture and resolution in dialectical behavior therapy for borderline personality disorder. *Journal of Personality Disorders, 32*(Suppl.), 115–128. https://doi.org/10.1521/pedi.2018.32.supp.115

Boritz, T., Barnhart, R., & McMain, S. F. (2016). The influence of posttraumatic stress disorder on treatment outcomes of patients with borderline personality disorder. *Journal of Personality Disorders, 30*(3), 395–407. https://doi.org/10.1521/pedi_2015_29_207

Borkovec, T. D., & Castonguay, L. G. (1998). What is the scientific meaning of empirically supported therapy? *Journal of Consulting and Clinical Psychology, 66*(1), 136–142. https://doi.org/10.1037/0022-006X.66.1.136

Bradley, M. M., & Lang, P. J. (1994). Measuring emotion: The self-assessment manikin and the semantic differential. *Journal of Behavior Therapy and Experimental Psychiatry, 25*(1), 49–59. https://doi.org/10.1016/0005-7916(94)90063-9

Brewster, B. (1882). Portfolio. *Yale Literary Magazine.* https://babel.hathitrust.org/cgi/pt?id=mdp.39015068303018&view=1up&seq=223&q1=theory%20and%20practice

Buchheim, A., & George, C. (2011). Attachment disorganization in borderline personality disorder and anxiety disorder. In J. Solomon & C. George (Eds.), *Disorganized attachment and caregiving* (pp. 343–382). Guilford Press.

Budge, S. L., Moore, J. T., Del Re, A. C., Wampold, B. E., Baardseth, T. P., & Nienhuis, J. B. (2013). The effectiveness of evidence-based treatments for personality disorders when comparing treatment-as-usual and bona fide treatments. *Clinical Psychology Review, 33*(8), 1057–1066. https://doi.org/10.1016/j.cpr.2013.08.003

Campbell, J. D., Trapnell, P. D., Heine, S. J., Katz, I. M., Lavallee, L. F., & Lehman, D. R. (1996). Self-concept clarity: Measurement, personality correlates, and cultural boundaries. *Journal of Personality and Social Psychology, 70*(1), 141–156. https://doi.org/10.1037/0022-3514.70.1.141

Carcione, A., Dimaggio, G., Conti, L., Nicolò, G., Fiore, D., Procacci, M., & Semerari, A. (2010). *Metacognition Assessment Scale (MAS) V.4.0. manual* [Unpublished manuscript].

Cardona, N. D., Southward, M. W., Furbish, K., Comeau, A., & Sauer-Zavala, S. (2021). Nomothetic and idiographic patterns of responses to emotions in borderline personality disorder. *Personality Disorders: Theory, Research, and Treatment, 12*(4), 354–364. https://doi.org/10.1037/per0000465

Carey, T. A., & Stiles, W. B. (2016). Some problems with randomized controlled trials and some viable alternatives. *Clinical Psychology and Psychotherapy, 23*(1), 87–95. https://doi.org/10.1002/cpp.1942

Carlson, E. B., Waelde, L. C., Palmieri, P. A., Macia, K. S., Smith, S. R., & McDade-Montez, E. (2018). Development and validation of the Dissociative Symptoms Scale. *Assessment, 25*(1), 84–98. https://doi.org/10.1177/1073191116645904

Cash, S. K., Hardy, G. E., Kellett, S., & Parry, G. (2014). Alliance ruptures and resolution during cognitive behaviour therapy with patients with borderline personality disorder. *Psychotherapy Research, 24*(2), 132–145. https://doi.org/10.1080/10503307.2013.838652

Caspar, F. (2018). Studying effects and process in psychotherapy for personality disorders. *Psychopathology, 1*(2), 141–148. https://doi.org/10.1159/000487895

Caspar, F. (2019). Plan analysis and the motive-oriented therapeutic relationship. In U. Kramer (Ed.), *Case formulation for personality disorders: Tailoring psychotherapy to the individual client* (pp. 265–290). Academic Press. https://doi.org/10.1016/B978-0-12-813521-1.00014-X

Caspar, F. (2022). Optimizing psychotherapy with plan analysis. In T. D. Eells (Ed.), *Handbook of psychotherapy case formulation* (3rd ed., pp. 209–251). Guilford Press.

Caspar, F., Silberschatz, G., Goldfried, M., & Watson, J. (2010). Similarities and differences in four views of David. *Journal of Psychotherapy Integration, 20*(1), 101–110. https://doi.org/10.1037/a0018886

Castonguay, L. G., & Beutler, L. E. (2006a). Principles of therapeutic change: A task force on participants, relationships, and techniques factors. *Journal of Clinical Psychology, 62*(6), 631–638. https://doi.org/10.1002/jclp.20256

Castonguay, L. G., & Beutler, L. E. (Eds.). (2006b). *Principles of therapeutic change that work*. Oxford University Press.

Castonguay, L. G., Constantino, M. J., & Beutler, L. E. (Eds.). (2019). *Principles of change: How psychotherapists implement research into practice*. Oxford University Press.

Castonguay, L. G., & Hill, C. E. (Eds.). (2017). *How and why are some therapists better than others? Understanding therapist effects*. American Psychological Association. https://doi.org/10.1037/0000034-000

Chanen, A., Sharp, C., Hoffman, P., & the Global Alliance for Prevention and Early Intervention for Borderline Personality Disorder. (2017). Prevention and early intervention for borderline personality disorder: A novel public health priority. *World Psychiatry, 16*(2), 215–216. https://doi.org/10.1002/wps.20429

Cheek, J. M., & Briggs, S. R. (2013). *Aspects of Identity Questionnaire (AIQ-IV)*. Measurement Instrument Database for the Social Sciences.

Chiesa, M., Luyten, P., & Fonagy, P. (2021). Two-year follow-up and changes in reflective functioning in specialist and nonspecialist treatment models for personality disorder. *Personality Disorders: Theory, Research and Treatment, 12*(3), 249–260. https://doi.org/10.1037/per0000464

Choi-Kain, L. W., Finch, E. F., Masland, S. R., Jenkins, J. A., & Unruh, B. T. (2017). What works in the treatment of borderline personality disorder. *Current Behavioral Neuroscience Reports, 4*(1), 21–30. https://doi.org/10.1007/s40473-017-0103-z

Clark, L. A., Cuthbert, B., Lewis-Fernández, R., Narrow, W. E., & Reed, G. M. (2017). Three approaches to understanding and classifying mental disorder: *ICD-11, DSM-5*, and the National Institute of Mental Health's research domain criteria (RDoC). *Psychological Science in the Public Interest, 18*(2), 72–145. https://doi.org/10.1177/1529100617727266

Clark, L. A., Nuzum, H., & Ro, E. (2018). Manifestations of personality impairment severity: Comorbidity, course/prognosis, psychosocial dysfunction, and 'borderline' personality features. *Current Opinion in Psychology, 21*, 117–121. https://doi.org/10.1016/j.copsyc.2017.12.004

Clarkin, J. F., Caligor, E., Stein, B., & Kernberg, O. F. (2007). *Structured Interview of Personality Organization* (STIPO). Personality Disorders Institute, Weill Medical College of Cornell University.

Clarkin, J. F., Levy, K. N., Lenzenweger, M. F., & Kernberg, O. F. (2007). Evaluating three treatments for borderline personality disorder: A multiwave study. *The American Journal of Psychiatry, 164*(6), 922–928. https://doi.org/10.1176/ajp.2007.164.6.922

Cloitre, M., Garvert, D. W., Weiss, B., Carlson, E. B., & Bryant, R. A. (2014). Distinguishing PTSD, complex PTSD and borderline personality disorder: A latent class analysis. *European Journal of Psychotraumatology, 5*(1), Article 25097. https://doi.org/10.3402/ejpt.v5.25097

Conners, C. K., Epstein, J. N., Angold, A., & Klaric, J. (2003). Continuous performance test performance in a normative epidemiological sample. *Journal of Abnormal Child Psychology, 31*, 555–562. https://doi.org/10.1023/A:1025457300409

Cristea, I. A., Gentili, C., Cotet, C. D., Palomba, D., Barbui, C., & Cuijpers, P. (2017). Efficacy of psychotherapies for borderline personality disorder: A systematic review and meta-analysis. *JAMA Psychiatry, 74*(4), 319–328. https://doi.org/10.1001/jamapsychiatry.2016.4287

Crits-Christoph, P., & Connolly Gibbons, M. B. (2021). Psychotherapy process-outcome research: Advances in understanding causal connections. In M. Barkham, W. Lutz, & L. G. Castonguay (Eds.), *Bergin and Garfield's handbook of psychotherapy and behavior change, 50th anniversary edition* (pp. 263–296). Wiley.

Cronbach, L. J. (1957). The two disciplines of scientific psychology. *American Psychologist, 12*(11), 631–684. https://doi.org/10.1037/h0043943

Cuijpers, P. (2019). Targets and outcomes of psychotherapies for mental disorders: An overview. *World Psychiatry, 18*(3), 276–285. https://doi.org/10.1002/wps.20661

Culina, I., Fiscalini, E., Martin Soelch, C., & Kramer, U. (2022). The first session matters: Therapist responsiveness and the therapeutic alliance in the treatment of borderline personality disorder. *Clinical Psychology and Psychotherapy, 30*(1), 131–140. https://doi.org/10.1002/cpp.2783

Davidson, K., Norrie, J., Tyrer, P., Gumley, A., Tata, P., Murray, H., & Palmer, S. (2006). The effectiveness of cognitive behavior therapy for borderline personality disorder: Results from the borderline personality disorder study of cognitive therapy (BOSCOT) trial. *Journal of Personality Disorders, 20*(5), 450–465. https://doi.org/10.1521/pedi.2006.20.5.450

De Meulemeester, C., Vansteelandt, K., Luyten, P., & Lowyck, B. (2018). Mentalizing as a mechanism of change in the treatment of patients with borderline personality disorder: A parallel process growth modeling approach. *Personality Disorders, 9*(1), 22–29. https://doi.org/10.1037/per0000256

Derogatis, L. R. (1975). *The Affects Balance Scale.* Clinical Psychometric Research.

Deutsch, H. (1942). Some forms of emotional disturbance and their relationship to schizophrenia. *The Psychoanalytic Quarterly, 11*(3), 301–321. https://doi.org/10.1080/21674086.1942.11925501

Dickey, C. C., McCarley, R. W., & Shenton, M. E. (2002). The brain in schizotypal personality disorder: A review of structural MRI and CT findings. *Harvard Review of Psychiatry, 10*(1), 1–15. https://doi.org/10.1080/10673220216201

Doss, B. D. (2004). Changing the way we study change in psychotherapy. *Clinical Psychology: Science and Practice, 11*(4), 368–386. https://doi.org/10.1093/clipsy.bph094

Drapeau, M., Perry, J. C., & Körner, A. (2012). Interpersonal patterns in borderline personality disorder. *Journal of Personality Disorders, 26*(4), 583–592. https://doi.org/10.1521/pedi.2012.26.4.583

Driessen, M., Wingenfeld, K., Rullkoetter, N., Mensebach, C., Woermann, F. G., Mertens, M., & Beblo, T. (2009). One-year functional magnetic resonance imaging follow-up study of neural activation during the recall of unresolved negative life events in borderline personality disorder. *Psychological Medicine, 39*(3), 507–516. https://doi.org/10.1017/S0033291708003358

Dziobek, I., Preissler, S., Grozdanovic, Z., Heuser, I., Heekeren, H. R., & Roepke, S. (2011). Neuronal correlates of altered empathy and social cognition in borderline personality disorder. *NeuroImage, 57*(2), 539–548. https://doi.org/10.1016/j.neuroimage.2011.05.005

Eells, T. D. (2022). *Handbook of psychotherapy case formulation* (3rd ed.). Guilford Press.

Ellison, W. D., Levy, K. N., Cain, N. M., Ansell, E. B., & Pincus, A. L. (2013). The impact of pathological narcissism on psychotherapy utilization, initial symptom severity, and early-treatment symptom change: A naturalistic investigation. *Journal of Personality Assessment, 95*(3), 291–300. https://doi.org/10.1080/00223891.2012.742904

Emmelkamp, P. M. G., Bouman, T. K., & Blaauw, E. (1994). Individualized versus standardized therapy: A comparative evaluation with obsessive compulsive patients. *Clinical Psychology & Psychotherapy, 1*(2), 95–100. https://doi.org/10.1002/cpp.5640010206

Erikson, E. H. (1950). *Childhood and society*. Norton.

Eubanks, C. F., Muran, J. C., & Safran, J. D. (2018). Alliance rupture repair: A meta-analysis. *Psychotherapy, 55*(4), 508–519. https://doi.org/10.1037/pst0000185

Eubanks, C. F., Wallner Samstag, L., & Muran, J. C. (2022). *Rupture and repair in psychotherapy: A critical process for change*. American Psychological Association. https://doi.org/10.1037/0000306-000

Euler, S., Dammann, G., Endtner, K., Leihener, F., Perroud, N. A., Reisch, T., Schmeck, K., Sollberger, D., Walter, M., & Kramer, U. (2018). Borderline-Störung: Behandlungsempfehlungen der SGPP [Borderline personality disorder: Treatment recommendations by the Swiss Society for Psychiatry and Psychotherapy (SGPP)]. *Swiss Archives of Neurology, Psychiatry and Psychotherapy, 169*(5), 134–142. https://doi.org/10.4414/sanp.2018.00598

Euler, S., Stalujanis, E., Allenbach, G., Kolly, S., de Roten, Y., Despland, J.-N., & Kramer, U. (2019). Dialectical behavior therapy skills training affects defense mechanisms in borderline personality disorder: An integrative approach of mechanisms in psychotherapy. *Psychotherapy Research, 29*(8), 1074–1085. https://doi.org/10.1080/10503307.2018.1497214

Fernandez-Alvarez, H., Clarkin, J. F., Del Carmen Salgueiro, M., & Critchfield, K. L. (2006). Participant factors in treating personality disorders. In L. G. Castonguay & L. E. Beutler (Eds.), *Principles of therapeutic change that work* (pp. 203–218). Oxford University Press.

Fertuck, E. A., Jekal, A., Song, I., Wyman, B., Morris, M. C., Wilson, S. T., Brodsky, B. S., & Stanley, B. (2009). Enhanced 'reading the mind in the eyes' in borderline personality disorder compared to healthy controls. *Psychological Medicine, 39*(12), 1979–1988. https://doi.org/10.1017/S003329170900600X

Fischer-Kern, M., Doering, S., Taubner, S., Hörz, S., Zimmermann, J., Rentrop, M., Schuster, P., Buchheim, P., & Buchheim, A. (2015). Transference-focused psychotherapy for borderline personality disorder: Change in reflective function. *The British Journal of Psychiatry, 207*(2), 173–174. https://doi.org/10.1192/bjp.bp.113.143842

Fisher, R. A. (1935). *The design of experiments*. Oliver and Boyde.

Fleeson, W. (2001). Toward a structure- and process-integrated view of personality: Traits as density distribution of states. *Journal of Personality and Social Psychology, 80*(6), 1011–1027. https://doi.org/10.1037/0022-3514.80.6.1011

Fleeson, W. (2004). Moving personality beyond the person-situation debate: The challenge and the opportunity of within-person variability. *Current Directions in Psychological Science, 13*(2), 83–87. https://doi.org/10.1111/j.0963-7214.2004.00280.x

Fleeson, W., Furr, R. M., Mneimne, M., & Arnold, E. M. (2019). Using basic personality process models to inform the personality disorders: Core momentary stressor-symptom contingencies as basic etiology. In D. B. Samuel & D. R.

Lynam (Eds.), *Using basic personality research to inform personality pathology* (pp. 73–93). Oxford University Press. https://doi.org/10.1093/med-psych/9780190227074.003.0004

Flückiger, C., Del Re, A. C., Wampold, B. E., & Horvath, A. O. (2018). The alliance in adult psychotherapy: A meta-analytic synthesis. *Psychotherapy, 55*(4), 316–340. https://doi.org/10.1037/pst0000172

Fonagy, P., & Bateman, A. (2006). Mechanisms of change in mentalization-based treatment of BPD. *Journal of Clinical Psychology, 62*(4), 411–430. https://doi.org/10.1002/jclp.20241

Fonagy, P., Luyten, P., & Bateman, A. (2015). Translation: Mentalizing as treatment target in borderline personality disorder. *Personality Disorders, 6*(4), 380–392. https://doi.org/10.1037/per0000113

Fonagy, P., Luyten, P., Moulton-Perkins, A., Lee, Y.-W., Warren, F., Howard, S., Ghinai, R., Fearon, P., & Lowyck, B. (2016). Development and validation of a self-report measure of mentalizing: The Reflective Functioning Questionnaire. *PLOS ONE, 11*(7), Article e0158678. https://doi.org/10.1371/journal.pone.0158678

Fonagy, P., Steele, M., Steele, H., & Target, M. (1998). *Reflexive-function manual: Version 5.0 for application to the adult attachment interview* [Unpublished manuscript]. University College, London.

Friedel, R. O., & Stahl, S. M. (2018). The fundamentals of brain neurotransmission. In C. Schmahl, K. Luan Phan, R. O. Friedel, & L. J. Siever (Eds.), *Neurobiology of personality disorders* (pp. 39–56). Oxford University Press.

Gaebel, W., & Falkai, P. (2009). *Behandlungsleitlinie Persönlichkeitsstörungen* [Treatment guide for personality disorders]. Steinkopff Verlag.

Ghaderi, A. (2006). Does individualization matter? A randomized trial of standardized (focused) versus individualized (broad) cognitive behavior therapy for bulimia nervosa. *Behaviour Research and Therapy, 44*(2), 273–288. https://doi.org/10.1016/j.brat.2005.02.004

Glaser, J.-P., Van Os, J., Thewissen, V., & Myin-Germeys, I. (2010). Psychotic reactivity in borderline personality disorder. *Acta Psychiatrica Scandinavica, 121*(2), 125–134. https://doi.org/10.1111/j.1600-0447.2009.01427.x

Goldfried, M. R. (1980). Toward the delineation of therapeutic change principles. *American Psychologist, 35*(11), 991–999. https://doi.org/10.1037/0003-066X.35.11.991

Goldfried, M. R. (2019). Obtaining consensus in psychotherapy: What holds us back? *American Psychologist, 74*(4), 484–496. https://doi.org/10.1037/amp0000365

Goldfried, M. R., Pachankis, J. E., & Goodwin, B. J. (2019). A history of psychotherapy integration. In J. C. Norcross & M. R. Goldfried (Eds.), *Handbook of psychotherapy integration* (3rd ed., pp. 28–63). Oxford University Press.

Goldfried, M. R., & Wolfe, B. E. (1998). Toward a more clinically valid approach to therapy research. *Journal of Consulting and Clinical Psychology, 66*(1), 143–150. https://doi.org/10.1037/0022-006X.66.1.143

Gratz, K. L., & Roemer, L. (2004). Multidimensional assessment of emotion regulation and dysregulation: Development, factor structure and initial validation in Emotion Regulation Scale. *Journal of Psychopathology and Behavioral Assessment, 26*(1), 41–54. https://doi.org/10.1023/B:JOBA.0000007455.08539.94

Grawe, K. (1998). *Psychologische Therapie* [Psychological therapy]. Hogrefe.

Greenberg, L. S. (1984). A task analysis of intrapersonal conflict resolution. In L. N. Rice & L. S. Greenberg (Eds.), *Patterns of change: Intensive analysis of psychotherapy process* (pp. 67–123). Guilford Press.

Greenberg, L. S. (2015). *Emotion-focused therapy: Coaching clients to work through their feelings* (2nd ed.). American Psychological Association. https://doi.org/10.1037/14692-000

Greenberg, L. S. (2019). Theory of functioning in emotion-focused therapy. In L. S. Greenberg & R. N. Goldman (Eds.), *Clinical handbook of emotion-focused therapy* (pp. 37–59). American Psychological Association. https://doi.org/10.1037/0000112-002

Greenberg, L. S., & Angus, L. (2003). The contributions of emotion processes to narrative change in psychotherapy: A dialectical constructivist approach. In L. Angus & J. McLeod (Eds.), *The handbook of narrative psychotherapy: Practice, theory and research* (pp. 331–349). SAGE.

Grenyer, B. F. S. (2013). Historical overview of pathological narcissism. In J. S. Ogrodniczuk (Ed.), *Understanding and treating pathological narcissism* (pp. 15–26). American Psychological Association. https://doi.org/10.1037/14041-001

Grilo, C. M., & Udo, T. (2021). Association of borderline personality disorder criteria with suicide attempts among US adults. *JAMA Network Open, 4*(5), Article e219389. https://doi.org/10.1001/jamanetworkopen.2021.9389

Gullestad, F. S., Johansen, M. S., Hoglend, P., Karterud, S., & Wilberg, T. (2013). Mentalization as a moderator of treatment effects: Findings from a randomized clinical trial for personality disorders. *Psychotherapy Research, 23*(6), 674–689. https://doi.org/10.1080/10503307.2012.684103

Gunderson, J. G., Fruzzetti, A., Unruh, B., & Choi-Kain, L. (2018). Competing theories of borderline personality disorder. *Journal of Personality Disorders, 32*(2), 148–167. https://doi.org/10.1521/pedi.2018.32.2.148

Gunderson, J. G., & Hoffman, P. (2016). *Beyond borderline: True stories of recovery from borderline personality disorder.* New Harbinger.

Gunderson, J. G., & Links, P. S. (2014). *Manual of good psychiatric management.* American Psychiatric Publishing.

Gunderson, J. G., Stout, R. L., McGlashan, T. H., Shea, M. T., Morey, L. C., Grilo, C. M., Zanarini, M. C., Yen, S., Markowitz, J. C., Sanislow, C., Ansell, E., Pinto, A., & Skodol, A. E. (2011). Ten-year course of borderline personality disorder: Psychopathology and function from the collaborative longitudinal personality disorder study. *Archives of General Psychiatry, 68*(8), 827–837. https://doi.org/10.1001/archgenpsychiatry.2011.37

Harned, M. S., Chapman, A. L., Dexter-Mazza, E. T., Murray, A., Comtois, K. A., & Linehan, M. M. (2008). Treating co-occurring Axis I disorders in recurrently suicidal women with borderline personality disorder: A 2-year randomized trial of dialectical behavior therapy versus community treatment by experts. *Journal of Consulting and Clinical Psychology*, *76*(6), 1068–1075. https://doi.org/10.1037/a0014044

Harpøth, T. S. D., Hepp, J., Trull, T. J., Bateman, A. W., Kongerslev, M. T., & Simonsen, E. (2021). Positive affect is associated with decreased symptom severity in the daily lives of individuals with borderline personality disorder. *Journal of Personality Disorders*, *35*(3), 355–372. https://doi.org/10.1521/pedi_2019_33_453

Hassan, N., & Will, H. (2006). Synthesizing diversity and pluralism in information systems: Forging a unique disciplinary subject matter for the information systems field. *Communications of the Association for Information Systems*, *17*(7), 152–180. https://doi.org/10.17705/1CAIS.01707

Hayes, S. C., Wilson, K. G., Gifford, E. V., Follette, V. M., & Strosahl, K. (1996). Experimental avoidance and behavioral disorders: A functional dimensional approach to diagnosis and treatment. *Journal of Consulting and Clinical Psychology*, *64*(6), 1152–1168. https://doi.org/10.1037/0022-006X.64.6.1152

Henry, J. D., Cowan, D. G., Lee, T., & Sachdev, P. S. (2015). Recent trends in testing social cognition. *Current Opinion in Psychiatry*, *28*(2), 133–140. https://doi.org/10.1097/YCO.0000000000000139

Herpertz, S. C. (2013). The social-cognitive basis of personality disorders: Commentary on the special issue. *Journal of Personality Disorders*, *27*(1), 113–124. https://doi.org/10.1521/pedi.2013.27.1.113

Herpertz, S. C., Matzke, B., Hillmann, K., Neukel, C., Mancke, F., Jaentsch, B., Schwenger, U., Honecker, H., Bullenkamp, R., Steinmann, S., Krauch, M., Bauer, S., Borzikowsky, C., Bertsch, K., & Dempfle, A. (2021). A mechanism-based group-psychotherapy approach to aggressive behaviour in borderline personality disorder: Findings from a cluster-randomised controlled trial. *BJPsych Open*, *7*(1), Article e17. https://doi.org/10.1192/bjo.2020.131

Herpertz, S. C., Nagy, K., Ueltzhöffer, K., Schmitt, R., Mancke, F., Schmahl, C., & Bertsch, K. (2017). Brain mechanisms underlying reactive aggression in borderline personality disorder—Sex matters. *Biological Psychiatry*, *82*(4), 257–266. https://doi.org/10.1016/j.biopsych.2017.02.1175

Hilsenroth, M. J., Holdwick, D. J., Castlebury, F. D., & Blais, M. A. (1998). The effects of *DSM-IV* cluster B personality disorder symptoms on the termination and continuation of psychotherapy. *Psychotherapy: Theory, Research, & Practice*, *35*(2), 163–176. https://doi.org/10.1037/h0087845

Hirsh, J. B., Quilty, L. C., Bagby, R. M., & McMain, S. F. (2012). The relationship between agreeableness and the development of the working alliance in patients with borderline personality disorder. *Journal of Personality Disorders*, *26*(4), 616–627. https://doi.org/10.1521/pedi.2012.26.4.616

Horowitz, L. M., Rosenberg, S. E., Baer, B. A., Ureño, G., & Villaseñor, V. S. (1988). Inventory of interpersonal problems: Psychometric properties and clinical applications. *Journal of Consulting and Clinical Psychology, 56*(6), 885–892. https://doi.org/10.1037/0022-006X.56.6.885

Huprich, S. K. (2020). Commentary on the Special Issue: Critical distinctions between vulnerable narcissism and depressive personalities [Special issue]. *Journal of Personality Disorders, 34*(Suppl.), 207–209. https://doi.org/10.1521/pedi.2020.34.supp.207

Hyman, S. E. (2010). The diagnosis of mental disorders: The problem of reification. *Annual Review of Clinical Psychology, 6*(1), 155–179. https://doi.org/10.1146/annurev.clinpsy.3.022806.091532

Jaspers, K. (1963). *General psychopathology*. John Hopkins University Press. (Original work published 1923)

Jorgensen, C. R. (2018). Identity. In W. J. Livesley & R. Larstone (Eds.), *Handbook of personality disorders: Theory, research and treatment* (pp. 107–122). Guilford Press.

Kao, G. S., & Thomas, H. M. (2010). Test review: C. Keith Conners *Conners 3rd edition* Toronto, Ontario, Canada: Multi-Health Systems, 2008. *Journal of Psychoeducational Assessment, 28*(6), 598–602. https://doi.org/10.1177/0734282909360011

Kaplan, B., Yazici Gulec, M., Gica, S., & Gulec, H. (2020). The association between neurocognitive functioning and clinical features of borderline personality disorder. *Brazilian Journal of Psychiatry, 42*(5), 503–509. https://doi.org/10.1590/1516-4446-2019-0752

Kazdin, A. E. (2009). Understanding how and why psychotherapy leads to change. *Psychotherapy Research, 19*(4–5), 418–428. https://doi.org/10.1080/10503300802448899

Keefe, J. R., Kim, T. T., DeRubeis, R. J., Streiner, D. L., Links, P. S., & McMain, S. F. (2020). Treatment selection in borderline personality disorder between dialectical behavior therapy and psychodynamic psychiatric management. *Psychological Medicine, 51*(11), 1829–1837. https://doi.org/10.1017/S0033291720000550

Keller, S., Stelmaszczyk, K., Kolly, S., de Roten, Y., Despland, J.-N., Caspar, F., Drapeau, M., & Kramer, U. (2018). Change in biased thinking in a treatment based on the motive-oriented therapeutic relationship for borderline personality disorder. *Journal of Personality Disorders, 32*(Suppl.), 75–92. https://doi.org/10.1521/pedi.2018.32.supp.75

Kernberg, O. (1967). Borderline personality organization. *Journal of the American Psychoanalytic Association, 15*(3), 641–685. https://doi.org/10.1177/000306516701500309

Kernberg, O. (1968). The treatment of patients with borderline personality organization. *The International Journal of Psychoanalysis, 49*(4), 600–619.

Kernberg, O. F. (1970). A psychoanalytic classification of character pathology. *Journal of the American Psychoanalytic Association, 18*(4), 800–822. Advance online publication. https://doi.org/10.1177/000306517001800403

Kernberg, O. F. (1975). *Borderline conditions and pathological narcissism*. Jason Aronson.

Kernberg, O. F. (1982). Self, ego, affects, and drives. *Journal of the American Psychoanalytic Association, 30*(4), 893–917. https://doi.org/10.1177/000306518203000404

Kernberg, O. F. (1984). *Severe personality disorders: Psychotherapeutic strategies*. Yale University Press.

Kernberg, O. F. (2005). Identity diffusion in severe personality disorders. In S. Strack (Ed.), *Handbook of personology and psychopathology* (pp. 39–49). Wiley.

Kernberg, O. F. (2006). Identity: Recent findings and clinical implications. *The Psychoanalytic Quarterly, 75*(4), 969–1004. https://doi.org/10.1002/j.2167-4086.2006.tb00065.x

Keuroghlian, A. S., Palmer, B. A., Choi-Kain, L. W., Borba, C. P., Links, P. S., & Gunderson, J. G. (2016). The effect of attending Good Psychiatric Management (GPM) workshops on attitudes toward patients with borderline personality disorder. *Journal of Personality Disorders, 30*(4), 567–576. https://doi.org/10.1521/pedi_2015_29_206

Kiesler, D. J., & Schmidt, J. A. (2006). *The Impact Message Inventory Circumplex (IMI-C) manual* [Unpublished manuscript]. Department of Psychology, University of Richmond.

King-Casas, B., Sharp, C., Lomax-Bream, L., Lohrenz, T., Fonagy, P., & Montague, P. R. (2008, August 8). The rupture and repair of cooperation in borderline personality disorder. *Science, 321*(5890), 806–810. https://doi.org/10.1126/science.1156902

Kivity, Y., Levy, K. N., Kelly, K. M., & Clarkin, J. F. (2021). In-session reflective functioning in psychotherapies for borderline personality disorder: The emotion regulatory role of reflective functioning. *Journal of Consulting and Clinical Psychology, 89*(9), 751–761. https://doi.org/10.1037/ccp0000674

Kivity, Y., Levy, K. N., Wasserman, R. H., Beeney, J. E., Meehan, K. B., & Clarkin, J. F. (2019). Conformity to prototypical therapeutic principles and its relation with change in reflective functioning in three treatments for borderline personality disorder. *Journal of Consulting and Clinical Psychology, 87*(11), 975–988. https://doi.org/10.1037/ccp0000445

Kleindienst, N., Bohus, M., Ludäscher, P., Limberger, M. F., Kuenkele, K., Ebner-Priemer, U. W., Chapman, A. L., Reicherzer, M., Stieglitz, R. D., & Schmahl, C. (2008). Motives for nonsuicidal self-injury among women with borderline personality disorder. *Journal of Nervous and Mental Disorders, 196*(3), 230–236. https://doi.org/10.1097/NMD.0b013e3181663026

Koerner, K. (2012). *Doing dialectical-behavior therapy: A practical guide*. Guilford Press.

Kohut, H. (1966). Forms and transformations of narcissism. *Journal of the American Psychoanalytic Association, 14*(2), 243–272. https://doi.org/10.1177/000306516601400201

Kraepelin, E. (1907). *Clinical psychiatry*. Macmillan.

Kramer, U. (2014). Observer-rated coping associated with borderline personality disorder: An exploratory study. *Clinical Psychology & Psychotherapy, 21*(3), 242–251. https://doi.org/10.1002/cpp.1832

Kramer, U. (2017). The role of coping change in borderline personality disorder: A process-outcome analysis on dialectical-behaviour skills training. *Clinical Psychology & Psychotherapy, 24*(2), 302–311. https://doi.org/10.1002/cpp.2017

Kramer, U. (2018). Mechanisms of change in treatments of personality disorders: Introduction to the Special Section. *Journal of Personality Disorders, 32*(Suppl.), 1–11. https://doi.org/10.1521/pedi.2018.32.supp.1

Kramer, U. (2019). *Case formulation for personality disorder: Tailoring psychotherapy to the individual client.* Academic Press.

Kramer, U. (2020). Individualizing psychotherapy research designs. *Journal of Psychotherapy Integration, 30*(3), 440–457. https://doi.org/10.1037/int0000160

Kramer, U. (2021). Therapist responsiveness in treatments for personality disorders. In J. Watson & H. Wiseman (Eds.), *The responsive psychotherapist* (pp. 237–255). American Psychological Association. https://doi.org/10.1037/0000240-012

Kramer, U., Beuchat, H., Grandjean, L., & Pascual-Leone, A. (2020). How personality disorders change in psychotherapy: A concise review of process. *Current Psychiatry Reports, 22*(8), Article 41. https://doi.org/10.1007/s11920-020-01162-3

Kramer, U., Beuchat, H., Grandjean, L., Seragnoli, F., Djillali, S., Choffat, C., George, E., Despland, J.-N., Kolly, S., & de Roten, Y. (2022). Lessening of the pervasiveness of interpersonal patterns in borderline personality disorder explains symptom decrease after treatment: A process analysis. *Journal of Clinical Psychology, 78*(5), 772–784. Advance online publication. https://doi.org/10.1002/jclp.23275

Kramer, U., Blanco Machinea, J., Grandjean, L., & Pascual-Leone, A. (2023, May 11–13). *Event-based assessment of emotional processing as mechanism of change in psychotherapy: An illustration* [Paper presentation]. Society for the Exploration of Psychotherapy Integration 39th Annual Meeting, Vancouver, BC, Canada.

Kramer, U., Eubanks, C. F., Bertsch, K., Herpertz, S. C., McMain, S., Mehlum, L., Renneberg, B., & Zimmermann, J. (2022). Future challenges in psychotherapy research for personality disorders. *Current Psychiatry Reports, 24*(11), 613–622. Advance online publication. https://doi.org/10.1007/s11920-022-01379-4

Kramer, U., & Golam, M. (2019). Cognitive heuristics in borderline personality disorder across treatment: A longitudinal non-parametric analysis. *Journal of Clinical Psychology, 75*(7), 1320–1331. https://doi.org/10.1002/jclp.22775

Kramer, U., Keller, S., Caspar, F., de Roten, Y., Despland, J.-N., & Kolly, S. (2017). Early change in coping strategies in responsive treatments for borderline personality disorder: A mediation analysis. *Journal of Consulting and Clinical Psychology, 85*(5), 530–535. https://doi.org/10.1037/ccp0000196

Kramer, U., Kolly, S., Berthoud, L., Keller, S., Preisig, M., Caspar, F., Berger, T., de Roten, Y., Marquet, P., & Despland, J.-N. (2014). Effects of motive-oriented therapeutic relationship in a ten-session general psychiatric treatment of borderline personality disorder: A randomized controlled trial. *Psychotherapy and Psychosomatics, 83*(3), 176–186. https://doi.org/10.1159/000358528

Kramer, U., Kolly, S., Maillard, P., Pascual-Leone, A., Samson, A. C., Schmitt, R., Bernini, A., Allenbach, G., Charbon, P., de Roten, Y., Conus, P., Despland, J. N., & Draganski, B. (2018). Change in emotional and theory of mind processing in borderline personality disorder: A pilot study. *Journal of Nervous and Mental Disease, 206*(12), 935–943. https://doi.org/10.1097/NMD.0000000000000905

Kramer, U., Pascual-Leone, A., Berthoud, L., de Roten, Y., Marquet, P., Kolly, S., Despland, J. N., & Page, D. (2016). Assertive anger mediates effects of dialectical behaviour-informed skills training for borderline personality disorder: A randomized controlled trial. *Clinical Psychology & Psychotherapy, 23*(3), 189–202. https://doi.org/10.1002/cpp.1956

Kramer, U., Pascual-Leone, A., Rohde, K. B., & Sachse, R. (2016). Emotional processing, interaction process, and outcome in clarification-oriented psychotherapy for personality disorders: A process-outcome analysis. *Journal of Personality Disorders, 30*(3), 373–394. https://doi.org/10.1521/pedi_2015_29_204

Kramer, U., Pascual-Leone, A., Rohde, K. B., & Sachse, R. (2018). The role of shame and self-compassion in psychotherapy for narcissistic personality disorder: An exploratory study. *Clinical Psychology & Psychotherapy, 25*(2), 272–282. https://doi.org/10.1002/cpp.2160

Kramer, U., Simonini, A., Rrustemi, E., Fellrath, R., Stucchi, K., Noseda, E., Martin Soelch, C., Blanco Machinea, J., Boritz, T., & Angus, L. (2023, June 21–24). *Emotion-informed narrative as mechanism of change in a brief treatment for borderline personality disorder* [Paper presentation]. Society for Psychotherapy Research 54th Annual Meeting, Dublin, Ireland.

Kramer, U., & Timulak, L. (2022). The emotional underpinnings of personality pathology: Implications for psychotherapy. *Clinical Psychology: Science and Practice, 29*(3), 275–286. Advance online publication. https://doi.org/10.1037/cps0000080

Krantz, L. H., McMain, S., & Kuo, J. R. (2018). The unique contribution of acceptance without judgment in predicting nonsuicidal self-injury after 20-weeks of dialectical behaviour therapy group skills training. *Behaviour Research and Therapy, 104*, 44–50. https://doi.org/10.1016/j.brat.2018.02.006

Krawitz, R. (2004). Borderline personality disorder: Attitudinal change following training. *The Australian and New Zealand Journal of Psychiatry, 38*(7), 554–559. https://doi.org/10.1080/j.1440-1614.2004.01409.x

Kretschmer, E. (1925). *Physique and character*. Harcourt Brace.

Krueger, R. F., Derringer, J., & Markon, K. (2013). *The Personality Inventory for DSM-5 brief form (PID-5-BF)*. American Psychiatric Association.

Krueger, R. F., Derringer, J., Markon, K. E., Watson, D., & Skodol, A. E. (2012). Initial construction of a maladaptive personality trait model and inventory for *DSM-5*. *Psychological Medicine, 42*(9), 1879–1890. https://doi.org/10.1017/S0033291711002674

Kuo, J. R., Fitzpatrick, S., Metcalfe, R. K., & McMain, S. (2016). A multi-method laboratory investigation of emotional reactivity and emotion regulation abilities in borderline personality disorder. *Journal of Behavior Therapy and Experimental Psychiatry, 50*, 52–60. https://doi.org/10.1016/j.jbtep.2015.05.002

Kuo, J. R., & Linehan, M. M. (2009). Disentangling emotion processes in borderline personality disorder: Physiological and self-reported assessment of biological vulnerability, baseline intensity, and reactivity to emotionally evocative stimuli. *Journal of Abnormal Psychology, 118*(3), 531–544. https://doi.org/10.1037/a0016392

Landelijke Stuurgroep Multidisciplinaire Richtlijnontwikkeling in de GGZ. (2008). *Multidisciplinaire richtlijn persoonlijkheidsstoornissen: Richtlijn voor de diagnostiek en behandeling van volwassen patiënten met een persoonlijkheidsstoornis* [Multidisciplinary directive personality disorders: Guideline for the diagnosis and treatment of adult patients with personality disorders]. Trimbos Instituut.

Lane, R. D., Ryan, L., Nadel, L., & Greenberg, L. (2015). Memory reconsolidation, emotional arousal, and the process of change in psychotherapy: New insights from brain science. *Behavioral and Brain Sciences, 38*, Article e1. Advance online publication. https://doi.org/10.1017/S0140525X14000041

Lane, R. D., Subic-Wrana, C., Greenberg, L. S., & Yovel, I. (2022). The role of enhanced emotional awareness in promoting change across psychotherapy modalities. *Journal of Psychotherapy Integration, 32*(2), 131–150. Advance online publication. https://doi.org/10.1037/int0000244

Lear, M. K., & Pepper, C. M. (2016). Self-concept clarity and emotion dysregulation in nonsuicidal self-injury. *Journal of Personality Disorders, 30*(6), 813–827. https://doi.org/10.1521/pedi_2015_29_232

Leary, M. R. (2013). *Need to Belong Scale (NTBS)* [Database record]. APA PsycTests. https://doi.org/10.1037/t27154-000

Lee, R., Fanning, J. R., & Coccaro, E. F. (2018). The clinical neuroscience of impulsive aggression. In C. Schmahl, K. Luan Phan, R. O. Friedel, & L. J. Siever (Eds.), *Neurobiology of Personality Disorders* (pp. 157–178). Oxford University Press.

Lee, R. M., Draper, M., & Lee, S. (2001). Social connectedness, dysfunctional interpersonal behaviors, and psychological distress: Testing a mediator model. *Journal of Counseling Psychology, 48*(3), 310–318. https://doi.org/10.1037/0022-0167.48.3.310

Levy, K. N., Beeney, J. E., Wasserman, R. H., & Clarkin, J. F. (2010). Conflict begets conflict: Executive control, mental state vacillations, and the therapeutic alliance in treatment of borderline personality disorder. *Psychotherapy Research, 20*(4), 413–422. https://doi.org/10.1080/10503301003636696

Levy, K. N., Ehrenthal, J. C., & Martin, J. A. (2022). Borderline personality disorder. In S. K. Huprich (Ed.), *Personality disorders and pathology: Integrating clinical assessment and practice in the* DSM-5 *and* ICD-11 *era* (pp. 353–373). American Psychological Association. https://doi.org/10.1037/0000310-016

Levy, K. N., & Ellison, W. D. (2022). The availability of training opportunities in personality disorders in American Psychological Association- and Psychological Clinical Science Accreditation System-accredited clinical and counseling psychology doctoral programs. *Training and Education in Professional Psychology*, *16*(4), 376–384. https://doi.org/10.1037/tep0000376

Levy, K. N., & Kelly, K. M. (2009). Sex differences in jealousy: A contribution from attachment theory. *Psychological Science*, *21*(2), 168–173. https://doi.org/10.1177/0956797609357708

Levy, K. N., Kivity, Y., & Yeomans, F. E. (2019). Transference-focused psychotherapy: Structural diagnosis as the basis for case formulation. In U. Kramer (Ed.), *Case formulation for personality disorders: Tailoring psychotherapy to the individual client* (pp. 19–40). Academic Press.

Levy, K. N., Meehan, K. B., Kelly, K. M., Reynoso, J. S., Weber, M., Clarkin, J. F., & Kernberg, O. F. (2006). Change in attachment patterns and reflective function in a randomized control trial of transference-focused psychotherapy for borderline personality disorder. *Journal of Consulting and Clinical Psychology*, *74*(6), 1027–1040. https://doi.org/10.1037/0022-006X.74.6.1027

Lewis, G., & Appleby, L. (1988). Personality disorder: The patients psychiatrists dislike. *The British Journal of Psychiatry*, *153*(1), 44–49. https://doi.org/10.1192/bjp.153.1.44

Lind, M., Sharp, C., & Dunlop, W. L. (2022). *Why, how*, and *when* to integrate narrative identity within dimensional approaches to personality disorders. *Journal of Personality Disorders*, *36*(4), 377–398. https://doi.org/10.1521/pedi_2012_35_540

Lind, M., Thomsen, D. K., Bøye, R., Heinskou, T., Simonsen, S., & Jørgensen, C. R. (2019). Personal and parents' life stories in patients with borderline personality disorder. *Scandinavian Journal of Psychology*, *60*(3), 231–242. https://doi.org/10.1111/sjop.12529

Linehan, M. M. (1993). *Cognitive-behavior therapy for borderline personality disorder*. Guilford Press.

Linehan, M. M. (2015). *DBT skills training manual*. Guilford Press.

Linehan, M. M., Armstrong, H. E., Suarez, A., Allmon, D., & Heard, H. L. (1991). Cognitive-behavioral treatment of chronically parasuicidal borderline patients. *Archives of General Psychiatry*, *48*(12), 1060–1064. https://doi.org/10.1001/archpsyc.1991.01810360024003

Linehan, M. M., Bohus, M., & Lynch, T. R. (2007). Dialectical behavior therapy for pervasive emotional dysregulation. In J. Gross (Ed.), *Handbook of emotional regulation* (pp. 581–605). Guilford Press.

Linehan, M. M., Korslund, K. E., Harned, M. S., Gallop, R., Lungu, A., Neacsiu, A. D., McDavid, J., Comtois, K. A., & Murray-Gregory, A. M. (2015). Dialectical-behavior therapy for high suicide risk in individuals with borderline personality disorder: A randomized controlled trial and component analysis. *JAMA Psychiatry*, *72*(5), 475–482. https://doi.org/10.1001/jamapsychiatry.2014.3039

Lis, S., Derish, N. E., & Perez-Rodriguez, M. M. (2018). Social cognition in personality disorders. In C. Schmahl, K. Luan Phan, R. O. Friedel, & L. J. Siever (Eds.), *Neurobiology of Personality Disorders* (pp. 179–206). Oxford University Press.

Livesley, W. J. (2003). Diagnostic dilemmas in classifying personality disorder. In K. A. Phillips, M. B. First, & H. A. Pincus (Eds.), *Advancing DSM: Dilemmas in psychiatric diagnosis* (pp. 153–189). American Psychiatric Association.

Livesley, W. J. (2018). Conceptual issues. In W. J. Livesley & R. Larstone (Eds.), *Handbook of personality disorders. Theory, Research, and Treatment* (pp. 3–24). Guilford Press.

Luborsky, L., & Crits-Christoph, P. (1998). *Understanding transference: The core conflictual relationship theme method.* American Psychological Association. https://doi.org/10.1037/10250-000

Luyten, P., & Fonagy, P. (2018). The neurobiology of attachment and mentalizing: A neurodevelopmental perspective. In C. Schmahl, K. Luan Phan, R. O. Friedel, & L. J. Siever (Eds.), *Neurobiology of personality disorders* (pp. 111–132). Oxford University Press.

MacNamara, A., & Phan, K. L. (2018). Neurocircuitry of affective, cognitive, and regulatory systems. In C. Schmahl, K. L. Phan, R. O. Friedel (Eds.), & L. J. Siever (Collaborator), *Neurobiology of personality disorders* (pp. 3–38). Oxford University Press.

Maillard, P., Dimaggio, G., Berthoud, L., de Roten, Y., Despland, J.-N., & Kramer, U. (2019). Metacognitive improvement and symptom change in a 3-month treatment for borderline personality disorder. *Psychology and Psychotherapy: Theory, Research and Practice, 93*(2), 309–325. https://doi.org/10.1111/papt.12219

Mancke, F., Schmitt, R., Winter, D., Niedtfeld, I., Herpertz, S. C., & Schmahl, C. (2018). Assessing the marks of change: How psychotherapy alters the brain structure in women with borderline personality disorder. *Journal of Psychiatry and Neurosciences, 43*(3), 171–181. https://doi.org/10.1503/jpn.170132

Marceau, E. M., Meuldijk, D., Townsend, M. L., Solowij, N., & Grenyer, B. F. S. (2018). Biomarker correlates of psychotherapy outcomes in borderline personality disorder: A systematic review. *Neuroscience and Biobehavioral Reviews, 94,* 166–178. https://doi.org/10.1016/j.neubiorev.2018.09.001

McCullough, J., Schramm, E., & Penberthy, J. K. (2014). *CBASP as a distinctive treatment for persistent depressive disorder.* Routledge. https://doi.org/10.4324/9781315743196

McHugh, C., & Balaratnasingam, S. (2018). Impulsivity in personality disorders: Current views and future directions. *Current Opinion in Psychiatry, 31*(1), 63–68. https://doi.org/10.1097/YCO.0000000000000383

McMain, S., Links, P. S., Guimond, T., Wnuk, S., Eynan, R., Bergmans, Y., & Warwar, S. (2013). An exploratory study of the relationship between changes in emotion and cognitive processes and treatment outcome in borderline personality disorder. *Psychotherapy Research, 23*(6), 658–673. https://doi.org/10.1080/10503307.2013.838653

McMain, S. F., Boritz, T. Z., & Leybman, M. J. (2015). Common strategies for cultivating a positive therapy relationship in the treatment of borderline personality disorder. *Journal of Psychotherapy Integration, 25*(1), 20–29. https://doi.org/10.1037/a0038768

McMain, S. F., Guimond, T., Streiner, D. L., Cardish, R. J., & Links, P. S. (2012). Dialectical behavior therapy compared with general psychiatric management for borderline personality disorder: Clinical outcomes and functioning over a 2-year follow-up. *The American Journal of Psychiatry, 169*(6), 650–661. https://doi.org/10.1176/appi.ajp.2012.11091416

McMain, S. F., Links, P. S., Gnam, W. H., Guimond, T., Cardish, R. J., Korman, L., & Streiner, D. L. (2009). A randomized trial of dialectical behavior therapy versus general psychiatric management for borderline personality disorder. *The American Journal of Psychiatry, 166*(12), 1365–1374. https://doi.org/10.1176/appi.ajp.2009.09010039

McMain, S. F., Pos, A. E., & Iwakabe, S. (2010). Facilitating emotion regulation: General principles for psychotherapy. *Psychotherapy Bulletin, 45*(3), 16–21.

Miller, C. E., Townsend, M. L., Day, N. J. S., & Grenyer, B. F. S. (2020). Measuring the shadow: A systematic review of chronic emptiness in borderline personality disorder. *PLOS ONE, 15*(7), Article e0233970. https://doi.org/10.1371/journal.pone.0233970

Mischel, W. (1973). Toward a cognitive social learning reconceptualization of personality. *Psychological Review, 80*(4), 252–283. https://doi.org/10.1037/h0035002

Möller, C., Karlgren, L., Sandell, A., Falkenström, F., & Philips, B. (2017). Mentalization-based therapy adherence and competence stimulates in-session mentalization in psychotherapy for borderline personality disorder with co-morbid substance dependence. *Psychotherapy Research, 27*(6), 749–765. https://doi.org/10.1080/10503307.2016.1158433

Morgan, S. L., & Winship, C. (2008). *Counterfactuals and causal inference. Methods and principles for social research.* Cambridge University Press.

Muran, J. C., & Eubanks, C. F. (2020). *Performance under pressure: Negotiating emotion, difference, and rupture.* American Psychological Association. https://doi.org/10.1037/0000182-000

National Health and Medical Research Council. (2012). *Clinical practice guideline for the management of borderline personality disorder.* https://www.nhmrc.gov.au/about-us/publications/clinical-practice-guideline-borderline-personality-disorder#block-views-block-file-attachments-content-block-1

National Institute for Health and Care Excellence. (2009). *Borderline personality disorder: Recognition and management.* https://www.nice.org.uk/guidance/cg78

Neacsiu, A. D., Rizvi, S. L., & Linehan, M. M. (2010). Dialectical behavior therapy skills use as a mediator and outcome of treatment for borderline personality disorder. *Behaviour Research and Therapy, 48*(9), 832–839. https://doi.org/10.1016/j.brat.2010.05.017

Neacsiu, A. D., Rizvi, S. L., Vitaliano, P. P., Lynch, T. R., & Linehan, M. M. (2010). The dialectical behavior therapy ways of coping checklist: Development and psychometric properties. *Journal of Clinical Psychology, 66*(6), 563–582. https://doi.org/10.1002/jclp.20685

Neumann, I. D. (2009). The advantage of social living: Brain neuropeptides mediate the beneficial consequences of sex and motherhood. *Frontiers in Neuroendocrinology, 30*(4), 483–496. https://doi.org/10.1016/j.yfrne.2009.04.012

New, A. S., Hazlett, E. A., Buchsbaum, M. S., Goodman, M., Mitelman, S. A., Newmark, R., Trisdorfer, R., Haznedar, M. M., Koenigsberg, H. W., Flory, J., & Siever, L. J. (2007). Amygdala-prefrontal disconnection in borderline personality disorder. *Neuropsychopharmacology, 32*(7), 1629–1640. https://doi.org/10.1038/sj.npp.1301283

Noll, L. K., Lewis, J., Zalewski, M., Martin, C. G., Roos, L., Musser, N., & Reinhardt, K. (2020). Initiating a DBT consultation team: Conceptual and practical considerations for training clinics. *Training and Education in Professional Psychology, 14*(3), 167–175. https://doi.org/10.1037/tep0000252

Norcross, J. C., & Goldfried, M. R. (2019). *Handbook of psychotherapy integration.* Oxford University Press.

Nuzum, H., Shapiro, J. L., & Clark, L. A. (2019). Affect, behavior, and cognition in personality and functioning: An item-content approach to clarifying empirical overlap. *Psychological Assessment, 31*(7), 905–912. https://doi.org/10.1037/pas0000712

Ochsner, K. N., & Gross, J. J. (2005). The cognitive control of emotion. *Trends in Cognitive Sciences, 9*(5), 242–249. https://doi.org/10.1016/j.tics.2005.03.010

O'Neill, A., D'Souza, A., Samson, A. C., Carballedo, A., Kerskens, C., & Frodl, T. (2015). Dysregulation between emotion and theory of mind networks in borderline personality disorder. *Psychiatry Research: Neuroimaging, 231*(1), 25–32. https://doi.org/10.1016/j.pscychresns.2014.11.002

O'Toole, S. K., Diddy, E., & Kent, M. (2012). Mindfulness and emotional well-being in women with borderline personality disorder. *Mindfulness, 3*(2), 117–123. https://doi.org/10.1007/s12671-011-0085-y

Pascual-Leone, A. (2018). How clients "change emotion with emotion": A programme of research on emotional processing. *Psychotherapy Research, 28*(2), 165–182. https://doi.org/10.1080/10503307.2017.1349350

Patton, J. H., Stanford, M. S., & Barratt, E. S. (1995). Factor structure of the Barratt Impulsiveness Scale. *Journal of Clinical Psychology, 51*(6), 768–774. https://doi.org/10.1002/1097-4679(199511)51:6<768::AID-JCLP2270510607>3.0.CO;2-1

Paul, G. L. (1967). Strategy of outcome research in psychotherapy. *Journal of Consulting Psychology, 31*(2), 109–118. https://doi.org/10.1037/h0024436

Pearls, J., Glymour, M., & Jewell, N. P. (2016). *Causal inference in statistics: A primer.* Wiley.

Pearls, J., & Mackenzie, D. (2020). *The book of why: The new science of cause and effects.* Penguin.

Perez, D. L., Vago, D. R., Pan, H., Root, J., Tuescher, O., Fuchs, B. H., Leung, L., Epstein, J., Cain, N. M., Clarkin, J. F., Lenzenweger, M. F., Kernberg, O. F., Levy, K. N., Silbersweig, D. A., & Stern, E. (2016). Frontolimbic neural circuit changes in emotional processing and inhibitory control associated with clinical improvement following transference-focused psychotherapy in borderline personality disorder. *Psychiatry and Clinical Neurosciences, 70*(1), 51–61. https://doi.org/10.1111/pcn.12357

Perez-Rodriguez, M. M., Derish, N., & New, A. (2014). The use of oxytocin in personality disorders: Rationale and current status. *Current Treatment Options in Psychiatry, 1*(4), 345–357. https://doi.org/10.1007/s40501-014-0026-1

Perry, J. C., Drapeau, M., & Dunkley, D. (2005). *The Coping Action Patterns Rating System.* McGill University.

Pos, A. E., & Paolone, D. A. (2019). Emotion-focused therapy for personality disorders. In L. S. Greenberg & R. N. Goldman (Eds.), *Clinical handbook of emotion-focused therapy* (pp. 381–402). American Psychological Association. https://doi.org/10.1037/0000112-017

Prochaska, J. O., & Norcross, J. C. (2014). *Systems of psychotherapy: A transtheoretical analysis* (8th ed.). Cengage.

Rice, L. N., & Greenberg, L. S. (1984). *Patterns of change: Intensive analysis of psychotherapy process.* Guilford Press.

Rizvi, S. L., Hughes, C. D., Hittman, A. D., & Oliviera, P. V. (2017). Can trainees effectively deliver dialectical behavior therapy for individuals with borderline personality disorder? Outcomes from a training clinic. *Journal of Clinical Psychology, 73*(12), 1599–1611. https://doi.org/10.1002/jclp.22467

Rogers, C. R. (1942). *Counseling and psychotherapy: Newer concepts in practice.* Houghton Mifflin.

Ronningstam, E. (2020). Introduction to the special issue on narcissistic personality disorder. *Journal of Personality Disorders, 34*(Special Issue, Suppl.), 1–5. https://doi.org/10.1521/pedi.2020.34.supp.1

Ronningstam, R. (2016). Pathological narcissism and narcissistic personality disorder: Recent research and clinical implications. *Current Behavioral Neuroscience Reports, 3*, 34–42. https://doi.org/10.1007/s40473-016-0060-y

Rosen, G. M., & Davison, G. C. (2003). Psychology should list empirically supported principles of change (ESPs) and not credential trademarked therapies or other treatment packages. *Behavior Modification, 27*(3), 300–312. https://doi.org/10.1177/0145445503027003003

Rosenberg, M. (1965). *Rosenberg Self-Esteem Scale (RSES)* [Database record]. APA PsycTests. https://doi.org/10.1037/t01038-000

Rudge, S., Feigenbaum, J. D., & Fonagy, P. (2020). Mechanisms of change in dialectical behaviour therapy and cognitive behaviour therapy for borderline personality disorder: A critical review of the literature. *Journal of Mental Health, 29*(1), 92–102. https://doi.org/10.1080/09638237.2017.1322185

Ruggero, C. J., Kotov, R., Hopwood, C. J., First, M., Clark, L. A., Skodol, A. E., Mullins-Sweatt, S. N., Patrick, C. J., Bach, B., Cicero, D. C., Docherty, A.,

Simms, L. J., Bagby, R. M., Krueger, R. F., Callahan, J. L., Chmielewski, M., Conway, C. C., De Clercq, B., Dornbach-Bender, A., . . . Zimmermann, J. (2019). Integrating the Hierarchical Taxonomy of Psychopathology (HiTOP) into clinical practice. *Journal of Consulting and Clinical Psychology, 87*(12), 1069–1084. https://doi.org/10.1037/ccp0000452

Russell, D., Peplau, L. A., & Ferguson, M. L. (1978). Developing a measure of loneliness. *Journal of Personality Assessment, 42*(3), 290–294. https://doi.org/10.1207/s15327752jpa4203_11

Sachse, R. (2020). *Personality disorders: A clarification-oriented psychotherapy treatment model*. Hogrefe.

Sachse, R., Schirm, S., & Kramer, U. (2015). *Klärungsorientierte Psychotherapie systematisch dokumentieren: Die Skalen zur Erfassung von Bearbeitung, Inhalt und Beziehung im Therapieprozess* (BIBS) [Systematic documentation of clarification-oriented psychotherapy: The scales to assess the process, content and relationship in psychotherapy]. Hogrefe. https://doi.org/10.1026/02654-000

Sadikaj, G., Moskowitz, D. S., Russell, J. J., Zuroff, D. C., & Paris, J. (2013). Quarrelsome behavior in borderline personality disorder: Influence of behavioral and affective reactivity to perceptions of others. *Journal of Abnormal Psychology, 122*(1), 195–207. https://doi.org/10.1037/a0030871

Sansone, R. A., Kay, J., & Anderson, J. L. (2013). Resident didactic education in borderline personality disorder: Is it sufficient? *Academic Psychiatry, 37*(4), 287–288. https://doi.org/10.1176/appi.ap.12110194

Santangelo, P., Bohus, M., & Ebner-Priemer, U. W. (2014). Ecological momentary assessment in borderline personality disorder: A review of recent findings and methodological challenges. *Journal of Personality Disorders, 28*(4), 555–576. https://doi.org/10.1521/pedi_2012_26_067

Sauer-Zavala, S., Bentley, K. H., & Wilner, J. G. (2016). Transdiagnostic treatment of borderline personality disorder and comorbid disorders: A clinical replication series. *Journal of Personality Disorders, 30*(1), 35–51. https://doi.org/10.1521/pedi_2015_29_179

Scala, J. W., Levy, K. N., Johnson, B. N., Kivity, Y., Ellison, W. D., Pincus, A. L., Wilson, S. J., & Newman, M. G. (2018). The role of negative affect and self-concept clarity in predicting self-injurious urges in borderline personality disorder using ecological momentary assessment. *Journal of Personality Disorders, 32*, 36–57. https://doi.org/10.1521/pedi.2018.32.supp.36

Schmitt, R., Winter, D., Niedtfeld, I., Herpertz, S. C., & Schmahl, C. (2016). Effects of psychotherapy on neuronal correlates of reappraisal in female patients with borderline personality disorder. *Biological Psychiatry: Cognitive Neuroscience and Neuroimaging, 1*(6), 548–557. https://doi.org/10.1016/j.bpsc.2016.07.003

Schnell, K., & Herpertz, S. C. (2007). Effects of dialectic-behavioral-therapy on the neural correlates of affective hyperarousal in borderline personality disorder. *Journal of Psychiatric Research, 41*(10), 837–847. https://doi.org/10.1016/j.jpsychires.2006.08.011

Schnell, K., & Herpertz, S. C. (2018). Emotion regulation and social cognition as functional targets of mechanism-based psychotherapy in major depression and comorbid personality pathology. *Journal of Personality Disorders, 32*(Suppl.), 12–35. https://doi.org/10.1521/pedi.2018.32.supp.12

Schulte, D., Künzel, R., Pepping, G., & Schulte Bahrenberg, T. (1992). Tailor-made versus standardized therapy of phobic patients. *Advances in Behaviour Research and Therapy, 14*(2), 67–92. https://doi.org/10.1016/0146-6402(92)90001-5

Schulze, L., Domes, G., Krüger, A., Berger, C., Fleischer, M., Prehn, K., Schmahl, C., Grossmann, A., Hauenstein, K., & Herpertz, S. C. (2011). Neuronal correlates of cognitive reappraisal in borderline patients with affective instability. *Biological Psychiatry, 69*(6), 564–573. https://doi.org/10.1016/j.biopsych.2010.10.025

Schulze, L., Schmahl, C., & Niedtfeld, I. (2016). Neural correlates of disturbed emotion processing in borderline personality disorder: A multimodal meta-analysis. *Biological Psychiatry, 79*(2), 97–106. https://doi.org/10.1016/j.biopsych.2015.03.027

Sebastian, A., Jung, P., Krause-Utz, A., Lieb, K., Schmahl, C., & Tüscher, O. (2014). Frontal dysfunctions of impulse control: A systematic review in borderline personality disorder and attention-deficit/hyperactivity disorder. *Frontiers in Human Neuroscience, 8.* https://doi.org/10.3389/fnhum.2014.00698

Shanks, C., Pfohl, B., Blum, N., & Black, D. W. (2011). Can negative attitudes toward patients with borderline personality disorder be changed? The effect of attending a STEPPS workshop. *Journal of Personality Disorders, 25*(6), 806–812. https://doi.org/10.1521/pedi.2011.25.6.806

Siever, L. J., & Weinstein, L. N. (2009). The neurobiology of personality disorders: Implications for psychoanalysis. *Journal of the American Psychoanalytic Association, 57*(2), 361–398. https://doi.org/10.1177/0003065109333502

Signer, S., Estermann Jansen, R., Sachse, R., Caspar, F., & Kramer, U. (2020). Social interaction patterns, therapist responsiveness and outcome in treatments for borderline personality disorder. *Psychology and Psychotherapy: Theory, Research and Practice, 93*(4), 705–722. https://doi.org/10.1111/papt.12254

Silberschatz, G. (2005). *Transformative relationships: The control-mastery theory of psychotherapy.* Routledge.

Silbersweig, D., Clarkin, J. F., Goldstein, M., Kernberg, O. F., Tuescher, O., Levy, K. N., Brendel, G., Pan, H., Beutel, M., Pavony, M. T., Epstein, J., Lenzenweger, M. F., Thomas, K. M., Posner, M. I., & Stern, E. (2007). Failure of frontolimbic inhibitory function in the context of negative emotion in borderline personality disorder. *The American Journal of Psychiatry, 164*(12), 1832–1841. https://doi.org/10.1176/appi.ajp.2007.06010126

Silvers, J. A., Insel, C., Powers, A., Franz, P., Helion, C., Martin, R. E., Weber, J., Mischel, W., Casey, B. J., & Ochsner, K. N. (2017). VlPFC-vmPFC-Amygdala interactions underlie age-related differences in cognitive regulation of emotion. *Cerebral Cortex, 27*(7), 3502–3514. https://doi.org/10.1093/cercor/bhw073

Simons, J. S., & Gaher, R. M. (2005). The Distress Tolerance Scale: Development and validation of a self-report measure. *Motivation and Emotion, 29*(2), 83–102. https://doi.org/10.1007/s11031-005-7955-3

Simonsen, S., Bateman, A., Bohus, M., Dalewijk, H. J., Doering, S., Kaera, A., Moran, P., Renneberg, B., Ribaudi, J. S., Taubner, S., Wilberg, T., & Mehlum, L. (2019). European guidelines for personality disorders: Past, present and future. *Borderline Personality Disorder and Emotion Dysregulation, 6*, Article 9. Advance online publication. https://doi.org/10.1186/s40479-019-0106-3

Skodol, A. E., First, M. B., Bender, D. S., & Oldham, J. M. (2018). *Structured Clinical Interview for the* DSM-5 *Alternative Model Personality Disorders (SCID-5-AMPD) Module II: Personality traits.* American Psychiatric Association.

Smith, R., Lane, R. D., Nadel, L., & Moutoussis, M. (2020). A computational neuroscience perspective on the change process in psychotherapy. In R. D. Lane & L. Nadel (Eds.), *Neuroscience of enduring change: Implications for psychotherapy* (pp. 395–432). Oxford University Press. https://doi.org/10.1093/oso/9780190881511.003.0015

Sonley, A. K. I., & Choi-Kain, L. W. (2021). *Good psychiatric management and dialectical-behavior therapy: A clinician's guide to integration and stepped care.* American Psychiatric Association.

Steger, M. F., Frazier, P., Oishi, S., & Kaler, M. (2006). The Meaning in Life Questionnaire: Assessing the presence of and search for meaning in life. *Journal of Counseling Psychology, 53*(1), 80–93. https://doi.org/10.1037/0022-0167.53.1.80

Steiner, T. G., Levy, K. N., Brandenburg, J. C., & Adams, R. B., Jr. (2021). In the mind of the beholder: Narcissism relates to a distorted and enhanced self-image. *Personality and Individual Differences, 173*, Article 110608. https://doi.org/10.1016/j.paid.2020.110608

Stern, A. (1938). Psychoanalytic investigation of and therapy in the borderline group of neuroses. *The Psychoanalytic Quarterly, 7*(4), 467–489. https://doi.org/10.1080/21674086.1938.11925367

Stiles, W. B. (2009). Responsiveness as an obstacle for psychotherapy outcome research: It's worse than you think. *Clinical Psychology: Science and Practice, 16*(1), 86–91. https://doi.org/10.1111/j.1468-2850.2009.01148.x

Stiles, W. B., Honos-Webb, L., & Surko, M. (1998). Responsiveness in psychotherapy. *Clinical Psychology: Science and Practice, 5*(4), 439–458. https://doi.org/10.1111/j.1468-2850.1998.tb00166.x

Storebø, O. J., Stoffers-Winterling, J. M., Völlm, B. A., Kongerslev, M. T., Mattivi, J. T., Jørgensen, M. S., Faltinsen, E., Todorovac, A., Sales, C. P., Callesen, H. E., Lieb, K., & Simonsen, E. (2020). Psychological therapies for people with borderline personality disorder. *Cochrane Database of Systematic Reviews.* Advance online publication. https://doi.org/10.1002/14651858.CD012955.pub2

Swift, J. K., & Greenberg, R. P. (2012). Premature discontinuation in adult psychotherapy: A meta-analysis. *Journal of Consulting and Clinical Psychology, 80*(4), 547–559. https://doi.org/10.1037/a0028226

Traynor, J., McMain, S., Labrish, C., & Ruocco, A. (2021). Pre-treatment neurocognition is associated with self harm outcomes in dialectical behaviour therapy for borderline personality disorder. *Biological Psychiatry, 89*(9), S129–S130. https://doi.org/10.1016/j.biopsych.2021.02.334

Unruh, B. T., & Gunderson, J. G. (2016). "Good enough" psychiatric residency training in borderline personality disorder: Challenges, choice points, and a model generalist curriculum. *Harvard Review of Psychiatry, 24*(5), 367–377. https://doi.org/10.1097/HRP.0000000000000119

U.S. Department of Health and Human Services. (2023). *PROMIS.* https://www.healthmeasures.net/explore-measurement-systems/promis

Waldinger, R. J., & Gunderson, J. G. (1987). *Effective psychotherapy with borderline patients: Case studies.* Macmillan.

Warwar, S. H., & Greenberg, L. S. (1999). *Client Emotional Arousal Scale—III* [Unpublished manuscript]. Department of Psychology, York University.

Watson, J. C., & Prosser, M. (2004). *Observer-rated Measure of Affect Regulation (O-MAR)* [Unpublished manuscript]. Ontario Institute for Studies in Education, University of Toronto.

Westen, D. (1985). *Self and society: Narcissism, collectivism, and the development of morals.* Cambridge University Press. https://doi.org/10.1017/CBO9780511598418

Whiteside, S. P., & Lynam, D. R. (2001). The Five Factor Model and impulsivity: Using a structural model of personality to understand impulsivity. *Personality and Individual Differences, 30*(4), 669–689. https://doi.org/10.1016/S0191-8869(00)00064-7

Widiger, T. A. (2018). Official classification systems. In W. J. Livesley & R. Larstone (Eds.), *Handbook of personality disorders: Theory, research and treatment* (2nd ed., pp. 47–71). Guilford Press.

Wierzbicki, M., & Pekarik, G. (1993). A meta-analysis of psychotherapy dropout. *Professional Psychology: Research and Practice, 24*(2), 190–195. https://doi.org/10.1037/0735-7028.24.2.190

World Health Organization. (2022). *International statistical classification of diseases and related health problems* (11th ed.). https://icd.who.int/

Yeomans, F. E., Clarkin, J. F., & Kernberg, O. F. (2015). *Transference-focused psychotherapy for borderline personality disorder: A clinical guide.* American Psychiatric Association.

Yeomans, F. E., Gutfreund, J., Selzer, M. A., Clarkin, J. F., Hull, J. W., & Smith, T. E. (1994). Factors related to drop-outs by borderline patients: Treatment contract and therapeutic alliance. *The Journal of Psychotherapy Practice and Research, 3*(1), 16–24.

Young, J. E. (2003). *Schematherapy.* Guilford Press.

Young, J. E., Klosko, J. S., & Weishaar, M. E. (2003). *Schema therapy: A practitioner's guide.* Guilford.

Zanarini, M. C. (2009). Psychotherapy of borderline personality disorder. *Acta Psychiatrica Scandinavica, 120*(5), 373–377. https://doi.org/10.1111/j.1600-0447.2009.01448.x

Zanarini, M. C. (2019). *In the fullness of time: Recovery from borderline personality disorder.* Oxford University Press.

Zanarini, M. C., Frankenburg, F. R., Reich, D. B., & Fitzmaurice, G. M. (2016). Fluidity of the subsyndromal phenomenology of borderline personality disorder over 16 years of prospective follow-up. *The American Journal of Psychiatry, 173*(7), 688–694. https://doi.org/10.1176/appi.ajp.2015.15081045

Zanarini, M. C., Gunderson, J. G., & Frankenburg, F. R. (1990). Cognitive features of borderline personality disorder. *The American Journal of Psychiatry, 147*(1), 57–63. https://doi.org/10.1176/ajp.147.1.57

Zanarini, M. C., Gunderson, J. G., Frankenburg, F. R., & Chauncey, D. L. (1989). The revised diagnostic interview for borderlines: Discriminating BPD from other axis II disorders. *Journal of Personality Disorders, 3*(1), 10–18. https://doi.org/10.1521/pedi.1989.3.1.10

Zeifman, R. J., Boritz, T., Barnhart, R., Labrish, C., & McMain, S. F. (2020). The independent roles of mindfulness and distress tolerance in treatment outcomes in dialectical behavior therapy skills training. *Personality Disorders, 11*(3), 181–190. https://doi.org/10.1037/per0000368

Zerbo, E., Cohen, S., Bielska, W., & Caligor, E. (2013). Transference-focused psychotherapy in the general psychiatry residency: A useful and applicable model for residents in acute clinical settings. *Journal of the American Academy of Psychoanalysis & Dynamic Psychiatry, 41*(1), 163–181. https://doi.org/10.1521/pdps.2013.41.1.163

Zimmermann, J., Woods, W. C., Ritter, S., Happel, M., Masuhr, O., Jaeger, U., Spitzer, C., & Wright, A. G. C. (2019). Integrating structure and dynamics in personality assessment: First steps toward the development and validation of a personality dynamics diary. *Psychological Assessment, 31*(4), 516–531. https://doi.org/10.1037/pas0000625

Index

About the Authors

Ueli Kramer, PhD, is a professor of psychiatry and psychotherapy, psychotherapy researcher and clinical psychotherapist, and director of the Institute of Psychotherapy at the Department of Psychiatry, University of Lausanne, Switzerland. He holds an adjunct appointment at the Department of Psychology, University of Windsor, Ontario, Canada. His research focuses on process and outcome in psychotherapy, in particular, the mechanisms of change in treatments of personality disorders and case formulation in personality disorders. Dr. Kramer has published over 180 scientific contributions and eight books. He is a broadly trained clinician, author, and editor, working from an integrative psychotherapy perspective. Dr. Kramer is a past president of the European chapter of the Society for Psychotherapy Research and current president of the European Society for the Study of Personality Disorders. Dr. Kramer's research has been supported by a number of grants and has been recognized by the Inger Salling Foundation, the Society for Psychotherapy Research, the Hamburg GePS Society for Personality Disorders, the AEMD Marina Picasso Foundation, and the Society for the Exploration of Psychotherapy Integration.

Kenneth N. Levy, PhD, is a tenured professor and associate director of clinical training, and served as interim codirector of the Psychological Clinic in the Department of Psychology at the Pennsylvania State University, where he directs the Laboratory for the Study of Personality, Psychopathology, and Psychotherapy. Dr. Levy also has a faculty appointment in the Department of Psychiatry at the Joan and Sanford I. Weill Medical College of Cornell University and is a senior fellow at Personality Disorders Institute. He is certified by the International Society for Transference-Focused Psychotherapy as a transference-focused psychotherapist, teacher, and supervisor. Dr. Levy's clinical and research interests are in the areas of attachment theory, personality disorders, and the psychotherapy process and outcomes. Dr. Levy has authored more than 200 articles and book chapters, as well as three books. Dr. Levy's work has led to awards and recognition from the American Psychological Association, the North American Society for the Study of Personality Disorders, the American Psychoanalytic Association, the National Alliance for Research in Schizophrenia and Depression, the Society for Psychotherapy Research, the Society for a Science of Clinical Psychology, the New York State and Connecticut State Psychological Associations, Cornell Medical College, the City University of New York, and Penn State University.

Shelley McMain, PhD, is the head of the Borderline Personality Disorder Clinic and a senior scientist at the Centre for Addiction and Mental Health in Toronto, Ontario, Canada. In addition, she is the director of the Division of Psychotherapy, Humanities, and Psychosocial Interventions at the University of Toronto and holds an associate professorship in the Department of Psychiatry at the University of Toronto. Dr. McMain was a past president of the Society for Psychotherapy Research, and she currently serves as the president of the Transitional Board of the World Federation of Dialectical Behaviour Therapy. Dr. McMain's clinical interests revolve around the areas of psychotherapy, dialectical behavior therapy, borderline personality disorder, emotion regulation, and the mechanisms of change. She has made significant contributions to the field, having authored over 90 published articles and book chapters and coauthored three books. These accomplishments have garnered recognition from various international professional associations, including the European Society for the Study of Personality Disorders, the American Psychoanalytic Association, International Studies, the International Society for the Improvement and Teaching of Dialectical Behavior Therapy, and the Personality Disorders Institute at New York Presbyterian Hospital and Weill Cornell Medical College.